OVERCOMING
MALE
INFERTILITY

OVERCOMING MALE INFERTILITY

Leslie R. Schover, Ph.D.,
and
Anthony J. Thomas Jr., M.D.

John Wiley & Sons, Inc.
New York • Chichester • Weinheim • Brisbane • Singapore • Toronto

Published by John Wiley & Sons, Inc.
Published simultaneously in Canada

The information contained in this book is not intended to serve as a replacement for
professional medical advice. Any use of the information in this book is at the reader's
discretion. The author and the publisher specifically disclaim any and all liability
arising directly or indirectly from the use or application of any information contained in this book. A health care professional should be consulted regarding your
specific situation.

Library of Congress Cataloging-in-Publication Data
Schover, Leslie R.
    Overcoming male infertility / Leslie R. Schover and Anthony J. Thomas
        p. cm.
    Includes bibliographical references and index.
    ISBN 0-471-24471-6 (paper : alk. paper)
    1. Infertility, Male—Popular works.   I. Thomas, Anthony J.   II. Title.

RC889.S375 2000
616.6'92—dc21   99-051353

Contents

PART TWO:
UNDERSTANDING MALE INFERTILITY:
CAUSES AND TREATMENTS

PART THREE:
COPING WITH MALE INFERTILITY

Illustrations

Acknowledgments

We hope that this book will be a helpful resource to the many men and women who have to confront male factor infertility. The most important debt of gratitude we can acknowledge is to the many patients who have taught us about courage and persistence; who have trusted us to help in the midst of their confusion and sadness; and who have rewarded us with their thanks as well as sharing their joyful baby pictures. Because we did not want to violate anyone's privacy, the case vignettes we have used as examples in this book reflect our experiences over the years, but are not actual individuals' histories.

We want to express our appreciation to a number of our colleagues: to Andrew Novick, M.D., chair of the Department of Urology of the Cleveland Clinic, for his support of this effort and of all our work together; to Ashok Agarwal, Ph.D., and his staff in our andrology laboratory, our partners in both patient care and research; to our teammates, the reproductive endocrinologists Tommaso Falcone, M.D., Jeffrey Goldberg, M.D., and Marjan Attaran, M.D.; and to the dedicated nurses who play such an important role in the lives of our infertility patients. We would like to thank Brian Clark, M.D., Ph.D., head of Medical Genetics at the Cleveland Clinic, and the genetic counselors Laurie Williams and Meagan Harris, for their valuable review and suggestions for chapter 7.

Most of all, we thank our spouses, Janie and Menachem, for their patience and inspiration while we took extra time from already busy schedules to write this book, and our children, for reminding us daily why all this effort to reproduce is so worthwhile.

Introduction

We decided to write this book after more than 10 years of working together at the Cleveland Clinic Foundation to help couples overcome infertility. Who are we? Anthony Thomas Jr. is a urologist who has specialized in male infertility for the past 20 years. He trains young urologists in this specialty area and has served as the president of the Society for the Study of Male Reproduction and as a member of the ethics committee of the American Society for Reproductive Medicine. Leslie Schover is a clinical psychologist who has worked with infertile couples and has researched the emotional aspects of infertility. We wanted to share some of our experience and knowledge with you.

Infertility treatment brings up not only medical and psychological issues, but ethical and spiritual dilemmas as well. We usually have a great time debating these topics, despite our very different backgrounds. Anthony Thomas is Lebanese American and a strong Catholic, while Leslie Schover is a Jewish feminist who has an easier time believing in space aliens than in God. Luckily we both share a good sense of humor and impatience with being "politically correct." We hope we can bring some lightness, along with empathy and a commitment to ethics, to leaven the pain of infertility for you, our readers.

HOW THIS BOOK CAN HELP YOU

This book provides information you need to understand the causes of men's fertility problems, find competent doctors who can help, and choose wisely among the treatment options you may be offered. It is geared for the couple with a male, or combined male and female, infertility problem. In addition to giving medical information, we also offer guidance in coping with the feelings and relationship issues that infertility brings. Some men who read this book may know they have a fertility problem, but are not in a relationship. Others may be married and in the midst of trying for a pregnancy.

In Part One, "Confronting Male Infertility," we discuss how couples often underestimate the rates of male infertility, how to find expert medical help, and what to expect during the evaluation process. We also describe the mechanics of sperm cell production and delivery. Part Two, "Understanding Male Infertility: Causes and Treatments," details the major syndromes that interfere with male infertility and the treatments available to overcome them. We describe assisted reproductive technology and donor insemination. In Part Three, "Coping with Male Infertility," we talk about ways that evolution may have shaped men's desire for children as well as discussing the women's point of view on infertility and ways a couple can become a team in coping with infertility treatment. We address spiritual and financial issues, adoption, living without children, and healing your sex life. At the end of the book is a resource section to help you find further information about male infertility, as well as a bibliography for readers who want to look up scientific material we mention and a glossary listing definitions for the medical terms we use.

We hope this book will be a helpful guide on your journey to overcoming male infertility.

Part One
Confronting Male Infertility

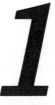

Male Infertility: Bumping into the Iceberg

Like a ship that hits a massive iceberg hiding beneath calm waters, it is usually a shock for a man to discover that he has a fertility problem. Throughout history, women have borne the burden of infertility. After all, their reproductive equipment is hidden, mysterious, and complex, while a man's organs seem to be right up front and simple. Most infertility specialists are gynecologists, and our culture focuses on a woman's anguish if she fails to become pregnant. The facts, however, differ from the stereotype. In the United States, about 40 percent of couples with infertility have a problem solely with the male partner. Another 20 percent of couples struggle with infertility problems on both the male and female sides. Only the remaining 40 percent of infertile couples have an exclusively female problem.

HOW COMMON IS MALE INFERTILITY?

Estimates for the 1990s suggest that around 5 million American women have fertility problems. By the year 2025, about 6.5 million women are expected to suffer infertility. We would expect a similar number of men to have trouble with fertility. In 1992, however, a Danish research group published a scientific paper that caught the world's attention. They observed a decline in men's sperm counts and quality over the past 50 years. Alarmed by their findings, these scientists speculated that industrial pollutants or other unknown factors were gradually decreasing men's fertility. The researchers feared that the same environmental changes were contributing to the growing rates of testicular cancer in industrialized countries and to an increasingly common birth defect known as *hypospadias,* in which the urinary tube opens on the underside of the baby's penis instead of at the very tip.

It is difficult to compare statistics on men's sperm counts across the last 50 years, since our ability to count sperm accurately has improved greatly with modern computerized technology. Researchers also debated about the right way to use statistics to understand the information available. In the United States and Europe, scientists searched their archives for records of men's sperm counts. Some studies agreed that sperm counts were declining, while others failed to find a difference across the years. The most recent consensus is that sperm counts have decreased in the United States from 1940 to 1990, although the average man's sperm count is still far above the levels needed for good fertility. We need a better understanding of why this change is occurring, and whether it has to do with pollution or other factors.

THE STIGMA OF MALE INFERTILITY

A barrier to getting help for a male infertility problem may be the negative feelings it brings. Of course men grieve when they are unable to have a child, just as women do. Men are often taught to cope with sadness by hiding it, however, and pretending that they are too tough to care. In their confusion and pain, some men deny the reality of their infertility, refusing to get medical help. In both the United States and western Europe, studies suggest that less than half of infertile couples seek treatment. Some men also see their fertility as part of their masculinity. A real man should father children effortlessly, like "sowing wild oats." Men worry that anyone knowing they have a low sperm count will also assume they are unable to have erections or intercourse. Some even confuse infertility with sexual orientation, and think that having a low sperm count may make a man homosexual. So let us be clear that infertility has no connections with a man's attraction to women, skill as a lover, success at football, or financial net worth; it is a medical problem with many different causes.

TREATMENTS THAT OFFER NEW HOPE

In the past several years, new developments in treating male infertility have made it possible for men to have their own genetic child when their only option used to be adoption or using sperm from a donor. The most major advance has been the success of in vitro fertilization using intra-cytoplasmic sperm injection, better known as IVF-ICSI. We discuss IVF-ICSI in detail in chapter 16, but it is mentioned so often in this book that we describe it briefly here.

In vitro fertilization (IVF) refers to combining egg and sperm out-side the human body, in a laboratory. In any type of IVF, the woman takes hormone injections to stimulate her ovaries to produce a number of ripe eggs. These are collected in a minor outpatient surgery and brought to the laboratory. Although the offspring of IVF have been called test tube babies, the process actually does not take place in a test tube, but rather in a small, flat plastic or glass dish known as a petri dish. One egg is placed in each dish along with thousands of sperm cells, in the hope that one will penetrate the egg and complete the process of fertilization. Any resulting *embryos* can be incubated in the laboratory for several days and then placed directly into the woman's uterus through her cervix. If more embryos develop than are needed for trans-fer, extras can be frozen, preserving them until they are thawed for a future replacement cycle.

Intracytoplasmic sperm injection (ICSI) is even more sophisticated. Once the eggs have been retrieved, the embryologist (a scientist expert in handling human eggs and embryos) uses a special, mechanized microscope to inject one sperm from the man directly into each egg. With IVF-ICSI, a man's semen quality no longer matters, as long as he can provide a few live and healthy sperm cells. Even if a man has no sperm cells in his semen, enough can often be gathered directly from the *epididymis* (sperm storage chambers at the top of each testicle) or even collected from a tissue sample from the testicle itself.

A number of other improvements in treating male infertility are dis-cussed in this book, including microscopic surgery to clear the sperm pathways and nonsurgical ways to repair a varicocele (a varicose vein in the scrotum). We also summarize new discoveries about genetic causes of male infertility.

You may be reading this book because you have already had a diagnosis of male infertility and want to learn more about what to do. Perhaps, however, you only have a suspicion something is wrong, but have not yet seen a doctor. The most crucial step in overcoming male infertility is to find an expert physician to guide your care. In the next chapter we suggest how to find the right infertility specialist and what to expect on your first visit.

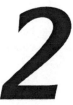

Getting Started with a Male Infertility Workup

Despite the fact that at least half of infertility is caused by problems on the man's side, finding expert care for male infertility can be frustrating. You can find a physician who specializes in treating male infertility, but you will need to be well-informed, assertive, and persistent. Some doctors still seem to believe the stereotype that infertility is a woman's problem, putting her through many expensive and painful tests without even ordering a semen analysis to rule out a fertility factor in the man.

Rita went to her gynecologist after 18 months of trying unsuccessfully to get pregnant. He told Rita he handled a lot of infertility. He had her keep temperature charts for several months, and although it looked like she was ovulating, he suggested trying clomiphene citrate (a frequently used fertility medication) for several cycles "just to give your ovaries a nudge." When a pregnancy still did not result, he performed a hysterosalpingogram, a very uncomfortable and expensive X ray of Rita's uterus and fallopian tubes. Since everything looked normal, he suggested a laparoscopy to check for endometriosis. That, too, was normal. Finally, in desperation, he sent Rita's husband, Danny, to a laboratory to have a semen analysis. Everyone was shocked when the results showed no sperm cells at all in Danny's semen.

Rita and Danny were more than shocked, however. They were angry. They had spent a year of their time and several thousand dollars out of their own pockets, since their insurance did not cover infertility-related medical care, when a simple laboratory test could have diagnosed their problem in a day.

One reason that men's problems often get overlooked is that more infertility specialists have training in finding and treating women's problems. There are over 10,000 members of the American Society for Reproductive Medicine, the major professional society in the United States for infertility specialists, but 90 percent are gynecologists and only 7 percent are urologists (the physician specialty that treats male infertility). Some gynecologists specialize in treating female infertility, taking an extra two years of advanced training and passing a board examination to be certified as reproductive endocrinologists. Urologists can also devote an extra year or two to advanced fellowship training in male infertility, but only a few of these programs are available and there is no certifying specialty examination. Other medical specialists may also be involved in treating male infertility. All can be called *andrologists* (specialists in studying men's sexual and reproductive function). Though some andrologists are physicians, others have a doctoral degree (Ph.D.) and are scientists who perform laboratory tests and conduct research.

Soon after the woman in a couple has seen her gynecologist for infertility, the man should have a semen analysis. Any physician can order the semen analysis, but you may want information on the qualifications of the laboratory performing it. Criteria to use in evaluating a laboratory, and other detailed information about the semen analysis, can be found in chapter 5. Even when a man's semen quality appears good, it does not guarantee his fertility. If all values in the semen analysis are within the range considered normal, however, further tests can proceed on the female side, unless there are specific reasons suggesting that a male problem needs further investigation.

If the semen analysis or other evidence suggests a male factor, it is best to find a specialist who deals a lot with male infertility. You may already be working with a gynecologist or an infertility clinic. Many infertility clinics have a specialist in male infertility on staff, or can recommend one in the local area. Sometimes, however, the gynecologist or reproductive endocrinologist will try to manage both male and female sides of infertility. Unless he or she is trained in evaluating male infertility, you might get shortchanged, missing out on a simpler or less expensive treatment that could solve your problem, or even missing a diagnosis, such as a testicular tumor, that impacts on your general health.

FINDING A MALE INFERTILITY SPECIALIST

Ideally, you would like to find a physician who has completed a special fellowship of one to two years in male infertility. Although doctors with this special training are not common, you may find one by calling the Department of Urology in a medical school or large hospital in your area and asking about the credentials of the physician on staff who takes care of male infertility. Other potential sources of information include your family doctor, who may know the reputations of infertility specialists in your local area, friends who have had treatment for infertility, or people active in your local chapter of Resolve, the support group for people with infertility (see "Resources").

Two national referral directories are also available to patients. The American Society for Reproductive Medicine (ASRM) has a list of its member physicians, their specialties, and their locations on its web site (see "Resources"). Just being in the directory does not ensure a physician's competence, but ASRM members have a special interest in reproduction and fertility and have to meet the society's ethical standards. Resolve also maintains a directory of physicians (see "Resources"). Resolve does have certain standards of training for including physicians on this list, and can give referrals for male infertility in a specific region.

No matter how you get the name of a potential male infertility specialist, you should do some research on his or her credentials. You can question the secretary in the physician's office or clinic, or call the medical board or local medical association in the nearest large city. Questions to ask include the following:

- Has the physician completed a special fellowship in male infertility?

- What percentage of the physician's practice is devoted to male infertility? (Most doctors do not spend the majority of their time on infertility, but the more specialized the physician, the better.)

- Does he or she belong to special professional organizations in the field, such as the American Urological Association and its subspecialty group, the Society for the Study of Male Reproduction; the American Society for Reproductive Medicine and its subspecialty group, the Society for Male Reproduction and Urology; or the American Andrology Association? Belonging to such societies *is no guarantee of a physician's competence,* but it does show a high level of interest in the male infertility field.

- Does the physician work with an assisted reproductive technology (ART) clinic that offers IVF-ICSI? This may become an important consideration.

- Does the physician work with a special andrology laboratory that offers high-quality semen analysis? The closer the communication between your doctor and the laboratory, the better.

- If the specialist is a urologist, does he or she perform microsurgical procedures to correct blockages of the sperm pathways? The surgical experience of the urologist is very important in these delicate operations. You may even want to know the surgeon's specific success rates if you are considering having a vasectomy reversal or other microsurgery performed.

- Does the physician do any research in male infertility? Many andrologists devote all their time to clinical work, but those who do some research are often at the forefront of their fields. Researchers usually work in a medical school or other specialized medical institute.

You may end up having an appointment with a doctor without being able to get this information in advance. In that case, you can politely and pleasantly request the same information from him or her. Explain that you are simply interested in getting the best care for your problem. You may want to inform the doctor at the beginning of the appointment that you have a few specific questions to ask. Although some doctors get huffy when patients ask about their credentials, someone who is truly expert should be glad to answer your questions. Infertility specialists are used to having well-informed patients, since those who seek help are typically educated and motivated couples who are paying for some or all of the medical care out of their pockets.

Of course, if you are lucky enough to have insurance coverage for diagnosis or treatment of infertility, your plan may restrict the doctors available to you. Even within a managed care organization or panel of preferred providers, however, you may have some choice over your specialist. Do all you can to make sure you see the best doctor for your problem.

WHAT TO EXPECT ON THE FIRST VISIT

Your first visit with an infertility specialist tells you a lot about the quality of care you will receive. An infertility evaluation should be thorough and wide-ranging, including both getting a health history and performing a physical examination.

Taking a History. The history, which may be taken by the doctor, a nurse or a physician's assistant, or by questionnaire, should include any childhood illnesses or surgeries you had that could affect your fertility (i.e., mumps that caused swelling of the testicles, hernia repair, bladder surgery, etc.); your history of major medical problems or surgeries as an adult; prescription medications you are taking; any work or hobbies that have exposed you to heavy metals, toxic chemicals, or chronic heat; your health habits such as smoking, use of alcohol, use of anabolic steroids for bodybuilding, use of recreational drugs, diet, and exercise; any knowledge of genetic problems in your family tree; and your current sexual practices. How long have you been having unprotected intercourse? How often do you have intercourse? Do you ejaculate within your partner's vagina? Have you been using any artificial lubricants for intercourse? Do you have intercourse on the most effective days of the cycle to promote a pregnancy? Are there any physical or sexual problems that might be interfering with effective intercourse? Have you ever caused a conception in the past (for example, with a different partner)?

The Physical Examination. A physical examination for infertility includes looking over your entire body. The doctor should check your overall appearance, including bodily proportions, body hair distribution, and general masculine traits. Your neck should be examined for an enlarged thyroid gland, and your chest for abnormal breast tissue enlargement. The abdomen is checked for increased liver size or other masses. Special attention is given to the genital area. The physician should examine your penis to make sure it is shaped normally and the opening of the urethra (urinary tube) is at the very tip. The doctor may ask if you have trouble getting erections. The physician will ask you to stand for a few minutes in a warm room before examining your testicles, so that he or she can spot abnormal veins, called varicoceles, that can interfere with fertility. The physician will gently examine the scrotum and the testicles, measuring their size and looking for signs of scarring or obstruction. Since 85 percent of the tissue in the testicle produces sperm cells, smaller testicles may indicate a fertility problem. The doctor will also check the cord leading to the testicle to identify a normal epididymis and vas deferens (see chapter 4). A rectal examination is often included to check the prostate and the seminal vesicles, glands which lie just in front of the rectum and contribute the fluids that make up the seminal plasma.

COMMUNICATION WITH YOUR SPECIALIST

Your specialist should give you some initial feedback on how things look. Many infertility specialists are happy to have your partner participate in the visit, at least for parts that just involve discussion. Some may not mind having her in the room for the examination, if you are comfortable with her presence. You should leave your specialist's office with some idea of the next steps in the diagnostic process and a feeling that you have someone on your side who cares about helping you.

THE SEMEN ANALYSIS

Before a diagnosis and plan for treatment can be made, however, the doctor needs to examine that very stuff of life—your semen. When men have fertility problems, there may be something awry with the number, activity, or shape of the sperm cells. Analyzing a sample of semen gives clues to the type and severity of the infertility. Unfortunately, there are a limited number of ways to get a sample of semen, and most of them involve some kind of sexual act that climaxes in *ejaculation*. Providing a semen sample is so awkward that men often delay infertility treatment or refuse completely to make an appointment. Therefore, we decided to confront this topic right away, just like you have to tackle it in real life.

3

They Want Me to Go into a Little Room and Do *What?*

You may find it humiliating that something could be wrong with your semen, but in order to have it analyzed, you have to do something that violates your privacy even more than an exam of your genitals or urinating into a specimen cup—you have to have an orgasm. Worse, you are usually asked to ejaculate by yourself through masturbation, often in a barren examining room located in a bustling medical clinic. It is not enough that you need to use your imagination or maybe some well-thumbed men's magazine to get in the mood, but you also need to follow medical instructions and catch the product of your labor in a sterile cup without missing a drop. Although you try not to think about it, outside that door is a laboratory technician who will probably be tapping her or his foot with impatience if you take more than five minutes to achieve this anticlimactic climax. Even if you have no trouble, you may encounter someone like the insensitive nurse who greeted one of our patients as he handed her his cup, "Wow! That was fast!" Do not close this book—or close the book on your infertility evaluation—yet, however. We have some suggestions that may make giving semen samples, if not a positive experience, at least a less dreaded one.

PLANNING AHEAD:
WHEN WAS YOUR LAST ORGASM?

"When was my last orgasm? That is a pretty personal question! Why does my doctor need to know?" No matter where you are giving a semen sample, infertility specialists usually recommend that you pay attention to the time since you last ejaculated. Any ejaculation, whether produced by your private self-touch, by partner caress, or during intercourse, uses up some of your stored sperm cells. If you have not ejaculated for a fairly long period, your semen may contain more sperm that are dead or have poor motility. The freshest sperm are the healthiest. On the other hand, if you have had a very recent climax, the amount of fluid you ejaculate and your sperm count may be lower than usual. It takes about 48 hours after the last ejaculation to restore a full contingent of mature sperm cells. Thus it is best to make sure you had your last ejaculation between two and three days before the day you collect your semen sample.

HOME DELIVERY

When the semen sample is needed for analysis only, rather than for an infertility treatment such as insemination of the woman or in vitro fertilization, you may be able to collect it in the privacy of your own home. The container you use to catch and transport your semen is important. Some types of containers can damage the sperm, so either get a special collection cup from the laboratory to take home, or use a clean, dry jar made of glass. The semen sample should preferably be collected through your own masturbation or from your partner's hand caressing. Collecting semen via oral sex or intercourse risks contaminating the sample with the bacteria that are naturally present in the mouth or the vagina. Some men have religious beliefs which make it crucial to collect a sample during intercourse, however. A few men also have great difficulty ejaculating except during intercourse. We discuss optimal methods for collecting sperm during intercourse a bit later in this chapter.

It is helpful to empty your bladder before you collect your semen sample, and to wash your hands. As long as your penis is clean and dry, you do not need to clean it in any special way. If you are not circumcised and tend to have whitish secretions build up under your foreskin, you may want to wash your penis before collecting the sample. Rinse well with water so no soap is left on your skin. Make sure your foreskin is pulled back at the moment of ejaculation. You should not use a lubricant such as petroleum jelly or K-Y when you stimulate your penis, because if sperm cells come in contact with a lubricant their motility (swimming power) may be reduced. It is important that you catch the whole ejaculate in the container, since the first few drops contain most of the sperm cells. The amount of fluid (volume) is also one of the factors examined in the semen analysis. The container is sized large enough to make an easy target. Do not fear! You are not supposed to fill it to the brim with semen! The average amount of fluid at ejaculation is only between one-half and one teaspoonful.

Since sperm cells begin to lose their motility right after ejaculation, you need to be able to get the semen sample to the laboratory in less than an hour. You also need to keep it at body temperature during the trip. We commonly suggest that a man (or the woman if she is the sperm courier) keep the container of semen warm by tucking it inside a waistband or a shirt pocket. Also avoid getting the sample too hot. One icy winter's day in Cleveland, one of our patients put her husband's semen sample in the glove compartment of her car. She did not realize that the heater would literally cook his sperm, so that they were all dead on arrival.

The advantage of producing a semen sample at home is obviously being spared the ordeal of masturbating at your doctor's office or a private room near the laboratory. The disadvantage is that the sample may lose some of its potency along the way, producing a less accurate test of your fertility or interfering with the success of treatment involving insemination.

I GAVE AT THE OFFICE!

If you collect your sample at your doctor's office or at a medical laboratory, you probably think that everyone in the waiting room knows why you are there. If the staff do not handle giving you your instructions discreetly, they may indeed figure it out. The one consolation is that most of the people in that waiting room have problems that are either similar to yours or even worse. Some clinics or laboratories have a deluxe collection room with a couch, a VCR, and a collection of erotic tapes and magazines. Others use a plain examination room or direct you to the men's room. You will probably not be surprised that a scientific study showed that men had a much easier time ejaculating when they were provided with an erotic video to watch, although their sperm counts and motility were no better than those of men who had to provide their own fantasy.

Here are some ways to make collection at the office easier.

- Many collection rooms are not well soundproofed. It can be very distracting to hear voices outside the door. Try bringing a personal tape player or radio so that you can use music to shut out the outside world and also to help you get in a more sexual mood.

- Bring your own erotic videotape (if a VCR is available in the collection room), book of stories, or magazine. Use them to get your sexual fantasies going.

- If you do not enjoy erotic pictures or stories, or if you find them unacceptable for ethical or religious reasons, try focusing your attention on pleasurable sensations in your body as you stimulate yourself. Another alternative is to remember a past sexual experience that was especially enjoyable. If you concentrate on the need to produce a semen sample, you may have difficulty reaching orgasm.

- If your partner is willing to help you, and you have a hard time using solo masturbation to reach orgasm, ask if she can come into the collection room with you. (Obviously this will only work if the hospital has a private room set aside for your collection.)

- Many men masturbate to orgasm occasionally even if they are happily married. Some men have not tried it since their teenage years, however. If you are a man who very rarely masturbates, practice at home before the crucial day, so that you know what kind of fantasies or stimulation works for you.

- If masturbation by hand is not comfortable for you, perhaps you would feel better about using a handheld vibrator to stimulate your penis. Vibrators are sold for body massage at stores that carry small appliances. Vibrators that are shaped like a wand with a vibrating head, and massagers that have a handle with snap-on attachments, both work well if you move them lightly over the sensitive areas of your penis. You could bring the vibrator to the hospital or doctor's office in a bag or briefcase. Some urologists and andrology laboratories have "industrial strength" vibrators that can be used to produce an ejaculation for men with spinal cord injuries. Once in a while, if a man is unable to reach orgasm when he needs to provide a sample, we will offer him this special vibrator to help.

COLLECTING THROUGH INTERCOURSE

A few men just cannot ejaculate except during intercourse. More commonly, however, a man requests to collect semen through sexual intercourse because his religion does not permit ejaculation outside of a woman's vagina. Most of the major world religions disapprove of sexual stimulation that is not designed to produce children. That is why masturbation is often considered taboo. On the other hand, when masturbation is prescribed by a doctor, not for sexual pleasure but to facilitate making a baby, many clergy will give their blessing in spite of usual religious laws. If you have questions about whether masturbation to collect semen for medical purposes is acceptable in your own religious framework, we suggest you consult a clergy person whom you respect.

Here are some views from major world religions on this issue, taken from available writings on the topic:

Religion	View on Semen Collection	Reason for This View
Orthodox Judaism	Masturbation is only acceptable as a last resort. Semen should be collected during intercourse using a collection condom (some rabbis specify the condom should be perforated to allow the possibility of ejaculation into the vagina). Laws that restrict intercourse to the times in a woman's menstrual cycle when she has been free of bleeding for at least seven days and has visited the ritual bath for purification should be observed.	Jewish law forbids "spilling one's seed" outside of the vagina and considers this a form of adultery. In general, however, conceiving a child is a duty and a blessing that supersedes most other laws governing sexuality.

continues

Religion	View on Semen Collection	Reason for This View
Conservative or Reform Judaism	Masturbation is acceptable as part of infertility treatment.	Conceiving a mutual genetic child for a married couple supersedes other religious concerns about masturbation.
Islam	Masturbation is not allowed as a sexual practice, but may be acceptable as a medical procedure for infertility treatment.	Procreation is a very important value. Infertility treatment is allowed, so long as it occurs within a marriage whose contract remains valid and preserves the mutual genetic heritage of the two parents.
Catholicism	Masturbation is not acceptable. Collecting sperm cells from the vas deferens or epididymis through a needle may be acceptable. Collecting semen through intercourse is acceptable if the condom is perforated, allowing the possibility of natural conception.	All conception should occur through sexual intercourse between spouses, uniting two fleshes into one in an act that symbolizes the sacred aspect of marriage and leaves open the possibility of conception.
Protestant Denominations	Most sanction masturbation to obtain semen for infertility treatment.	Evangelical churches may ban masturbation based on direct biblical sources such as those used by Orthodox Jewish or Roman Catholic scholars.

If you need to collect semen during intercourse, ask your doctor for a special collection condom made out of silicone. Condoms made out of latex rubber or lambskin will not preserve your semen sample properly. If your religious beliefs require that the condom have a perforation, it is best to make a very small pinhole as close to the open end of the condom as possible. A sample collected during intercourse may be good enough for diagnostic tests, but if you and your wife are collecting semen for a procedure such as intrauterine insemination (IUI) or in vitro fertilization (IVF), using a collection condom can result in contamination from bacteria and cells from the skin. This could interfere with the fertilization process. It may help to maximize cleanliness by washing your penis with a mild soap before intercourse. Rinse it all off carefully, using lots of water.

Some silicone condoms have a reservoir for the semen at the tip. If yours does not, pinch about an inch at the tip to create a reservoir space before you roll the condom on. As soon as you ejaculate during intercourse, withdraw your penis, holding the condom around the base of your penis with your hand to prevent leakage. Take off the condom slowly and gently, with your penis pointed at the floor to avoid spilling any of the semen. Wrap a twist tie around the open end of the condom to seal it, and put it inside a sterile container, ready to be transported to the laboratory.

Paradoxically, several studies have found that men's sperm counts and motility are better in samples collected during intercourse compared to those obtained with masturbation. This has held especially true for men whose sperm counts or motility were lower than normal. Thus some centers have encouraged semen collection through intercourse for infertility treatments such as intrauterine insemination, despite the concerns about contamination.

WHAT IF YOU DO NOT EJACULATE SEMEN?

Some men have fertility problems, at least in part, because they have "dry ejaculations" in which no semen spurts out of the penis. This condition can occur in some men who have diabetes, some who had surgery on certain parts of the bladder as children, or men who have had a few specific types of cancer treatment (see chapter 14). If a man's testicles produce sperm cells, there are a number of ways to retrieve sperm for diagnosis or fertility treatment, even if the man does not ejaculate. These new methods will be discussed in detail in chapters 13 and 16.

Now that you know what is involved in giving a semen sample, you are probably curious about the information that is in the report the laboratory sends to your doctor. Before we can explain the semen analysis, however, you need to understand the amazing process of sperm manufacture.

4

Your Baby-Making Machinery: An Owner's Manual

To understand a man's fertility, you need to know the answers to some basic questions: How are sperm cells made? What controls sperm production? How do the basic parts of a man's reproductive system fit together, and what does each part do? How does the sperm get to the egg? What happens when the sperm and the egg meet? This chapter will try to answer these questions without using too much medical jargon.

THE BASIC EQUIPMENT

As you can see from the illustration on page 24, a man's reproductive system includes two testicles where sperm are produced; an epididymis where sperm are stored and mature at the upper, back area of each testicle; two *vas deferens,* tubes connecting the epididymis with the ejaculatory ducts; two *seminal vesicles,* glands that produce most of the fluid in semen; one *prostate* gland, which contributes important chemicals to the semen; and the *bulbourethral glands,* which produce a few drops of fluid that lubricates and prepares the *urethra,* the tube running the length of the penis, for passage of urine or semen for ejaculation.

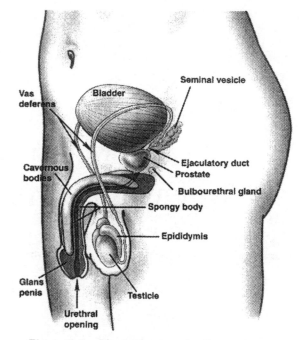

Figure 4.1   The male reproductive system

The Testicles. The testicles contain several important types of cells, each with a highly specialized job. The cells either contribute to making sperm cells or to manufacturing the hormone testosterone. Indeed, these two jobs are related, since sperm production needs testosterone to proceed.

There are many types of cells inside the testicle, but in order to understand the cycle of sperm production, you mainly need to know about the three most important types:

- Leydig cells
- Sertoli cells
- spermatogonia

The first two types of cells were named for the men who discovered and described them—Franz von Leydig and Enrico Sertoli. The term "spermatogonia" comes from the Greek words meaning "seed" and "generation." We will describe each type of cell in some detail, but first you need to picture the layout of a testicle (see diagram on page 25). The illustration should help.

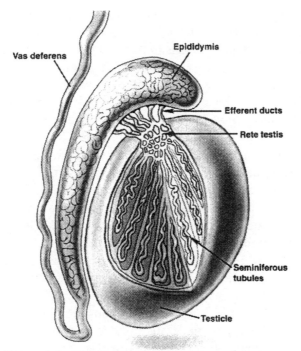

Figure 4.2   The testicle and its system of ducts

The interior of each testicle is normally filled by little tubes called *seminiferous tubules,* in which the actual manufacture of sperm takes place. If you could somehow unwind all of the seminiferous tubules and place them end to end, their total length would be hundreds of feet. In the testicle, however, they are compressed tightly beneath a thick, strong covering of tissue called the *tunica albuginea.* Inside each seminiferous tubule is an entire sperm cell factory unit. Although the same product is being made throughout the length of the tubule, at any one time different areas are producing sperm cells of varying ripeness, or maturity. Sperm production involves a series of repeating cycles. Sperm cells must go through a series of stages before they are finally mature and capable of fertilizing an egg.

The *Leydig cells* are located outside of the seminiferous tubules. Present in an immature form even before birth, they produce *testosterone.* Often called the male sex hormone, testosterone actually plays many roles. Before birth, it helps to guide the development of the male reproductive organs in the *fetus.* Soon after a boy is born, the Leydig cells produce a surge of testosterone that is thought to add the finishing touches to the unique male organization of the brain (perhaps including the famous tendencies to leave the toilet seat up and never ask for directions when lost). This spurt of hormones may also prepare the prostate and other reproductive organs to respond to testosterone at puberty. As a boy approaches his early teens, the testicles again begin producing higher levels of testosterone, leading to the bodily changes of manhood, including beard and body hair growth, growth of the penis, and deepening of the voice. These higher levels of testosterone also help to trigger sperm cell production. For the rest of a man's life, testosterone acts in his brain to promote desire for sex and helps men achieve and maintain erections. Some men who do not produce sperm cells still can make normal amounts of testosterone, however, allowing all the other male functions to occur. The Leydig cells only make testosterone if they receive a hormonal message from the pituitary gland that more of this hormone is needed, as we discuss shortly.

The *Sertoli cells* are perhaps the most unique cell type in the testicle, and have fascinated scientists interested in reproduction. When Enrico Sertoli first described them in 1865, he called them nurse cells, recognizing their role in guiding, directing, and protecting the formation of sperm in the seminiferous tubules. Sertoli cells form a lining in each seminiferous tubule, creating a barrier between the bloodstream and the sperm-producing units. This makes a perfect environment for sperm cell production and maturation. The tight barrier also prevents the body's immune system from reacting to the sperm cells. As we explain in chapter 9, when immune cells come into contact with sperm, they may form antibodies that interfere with sperm function. The Sertoli cells literally nurse sperm cells to maturity, supplying some of the crucial chemicals that sperm cells need in order to develop. Now we discuss the third type of cells, spermatogonia.

Sperm Cell Production. When the male fetus develops, a group of specialized cells migrates to the scrotum. They become the *spermatogonia (parent cells)* that will begin to produce ripe sperm cells at the time of a boy's puberty and will continue for the rest of his life. This is one of the many ways that men and women differ in their reproductive systems. When a female is born, her tiny, undeveloped ovaries contain all the egg cells she will ever have. When she reaches puberty and begins to menstruate, an egg (ovum) ripens each month. By the time a woman reaches her late 40s or early 50s, her egg supply has been depleted and she goes through her menopause, or change of life.

Males, on the other hand, are born without any sperm cells. They only have cells with the potential to form sperm. When a boy reaches

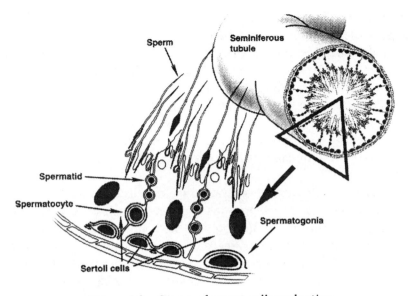

Figure 4.3   Stages of sperm cell production

puberty, the same hormones from the pituitary gland that stimulate a woman's menstrual cycles start the male process of sperm maturation. A man, however, may continue to produce sperm all his life, without ever using up his renewable supply. If he remains relatively healthy, sperm will always be present in his semen, even if he reaches his 80s or 90s.

Another difference between men and women (and there are certainly plenty!) is that in only one month an egg fully matures and is released, but it takes about three months to form, mature, and release sperm. This explains why it takes so long to see a positive change in a man's semen quality if he undergoes a treatment designed to improve his sperm production.

The illustration above shows the steps of sperm cell production inside the seminiferous tubules. In step 1 of the sperm production cycle, the parent cells (spermatogonia) each divide into two new, round cells. These duplicated cells will continue to grow and divide, but the parent cell will remain in its original state, always ready to make new copies of itself.

Like all other body cells, the parent cells and each of the two new copies have exactly 46 *chromosomes*. These chromosomes are tiny rod-shaped structures made up of *DNA (deoxyribonucleic acid)*, the genetic building code of living creatures. Chains of DNA form into genes, nature's blueprint. Within its 46 chromosomes, each cell has all the genes needed to build a complete human being. The 46 chromosomes are contained in the *nucleus,* or central structure of each cell, and actually form 23 pairs. Twenty-two of the pairs match, although each paired chromosome carries slightly different versions of the same genes (for example, a gene for blue eyes on one member of a pair, and one for brown eyes on the matching chromosome). The last pair of chromosomes includes the X and the Y, called the "sex chromosomes" because they determine a human being's gender. A female has two Xs and a male has an X and a Y.

In step 2, as the second generation sperm cells continue to divide, a special process, called *meiosis,* takes place. In meiosis, the chromosomes pair up during cell division, but then only one member of each pair enters each of the two new cells. These cells, called *spermatocytes,* contain only 23 chromosomes. During meiosis, the genes shuffle around somewhat between the paired chromosomes, so that each spermatocyte contains a unique combination of genes. And of course, each spermatocyte either contains just one X or one Y sex chromosome. Since the egg from the mother always contributes one X chromosome during fertilization, it is the sperm from the father that determines the sex of his future children.

After another cell division, the maturing sperm cell is called a *spermatid.* It still does not have the tadpole look of a mature sperm cell. Next the spermatid must lighten its load, losing most of the fluid, called *cytoplasm,* that surrounds the cell's nucleus. The spermatid also develops a whiplike tail called a *flagellum,* to help it swim, and an *acrosomal cap,* a helmet that covers about two-thirds of the sperm head. The acrosomal cap contains special enzymes that can drill a tiny hole in the shell surrounding the egg, allowing the sperm to penetrate and fertilization to occur. Now the spermatid has developed into a sperm cell. But it is not yet finished.

The Sperm Matures. Sperm cells are pushed along through the centers of the seminiferous tubules to a small cluster of tubes called the *rete testis.* From here they move out of the comfortable, protected testicle, through more tiny tubes to gather in the epididymis, lying just outside of each testicle. The epididymis serves as a "halfway house" for the sperm. Here, the sperm cells mature even further, gaining their ability to swim vigorously and survive in the cold, cruel world of the female's reproductive system.

Although each epididymis appears to be only about 3 by ½ by ½ inch in size, it is in reality a twisted, tortuous tube that would measure about 15 feet if extended to full length. Depending on how often a man ejaculates, sperm may spend from two to six days in transit in the epididymis before they reach the vas deferens and finally mix with the seminal fluid during ejaculation. The final stage of maturation, called *capacitation*, occurs not in the man's body, but in the woman's cervix. Capacitated sperm can swim faster and have undergone changes that help them bind to the shell around the egg.

WHAT IS SEMEN?

At the moment before outward ejaculation takes place, a mixture of semen and sperm comes through the ejaculatory ducts, passing through the prostate gland to the upper urethra. Semen contains ripe sperm cells that have just traveled through the vas deferens, as well as fluid from the prostate gland and the seminal vesicles. An average ejaculate contains between 0.5 and 1 teaspoon (1 teaspoon is 5.0 milliliters of fluid). The prostate gland contributes about a quarter of that fluid mix (0.5 to 1.0 ml), containing chemicals that will make the semen liquefy after ejaculation. The seminal vesicles (pouchlike glands that sit behind the urinary bladder) secrete about 1.5 to 5.0 ml of liquid. Fluid from the prostate and the seminal vesicles combined accounts for more than 90 percent of the ejaculate. The seminal vesicles are the only part of the body that produces fructose, a sugar that will nourish sperm cells and give them the energy for their long swim to the egg. The seminal vesicles also produce other substances that sperm need to survive and function once they enter the vagina.

Semen acts as a buffer to protect the sperm from hostile, outside influences on their journey through the woman's genital pathways. In order for a woman to maintain a healthy vaginal environment, her body produces mildly acidic fluids. If sperm came into contact with the vaginal surface without the protection of semen, they would quickly be immobilized. After ejaculation, however, healthy sperm quickly swim up to enter the more welcoming alkaline (opposite of acidic) mucus that coats the woman's cervix at the time of ovulation.

When a man is very sexually excited, a few drops of clear fluid may appear at the tip of his penis before he actually ejaculates. This fluid is produced by the bulbourethral glands. It appears to lubricate and clean

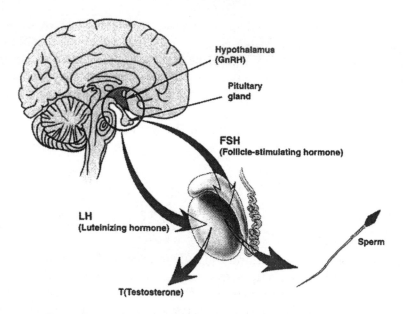

Figure 4.4   The brain-testicular hormone feedback cycle

out the urethra to prepare for the actual semen that is about to pass through.

THE BRAIN'S CONTROL SYSTEM

Although some women joke that a man's brains are controlled by his genital area, in reality it is the testicles that are controlled by the brain. The *hypothalamus,* an area deep inside the brain, produces a messenger chemical called *gonadotropin-releasing hormone* (GnRH). This chemical is sent directly into a small gland in the lower middle part of the brain, the *pituitary.* The pituitary responds by producing *luteinizing hormone* (LH) and *follicle-stimulating hormone* (FSH). Luteinizing hormone and FSH travel in the bloodstream to the testicles. There, LH tells the Leydig cells to produce testosterone. Follicle-stimulating hormone activates the Sertoli cells and keeps sperm cell production going. The hypothalamus, in turn, gets chemical feedback through the bloodstream about the levels of testosterone and sperm cells being produced.

If all is balanced, the hypothalamus may take a rest. If there is a lag in producing testosterone or sperm cells, the hypothalamus pumps out more GnRH, and the pituitary in turn revs up LH and FSH to compensate, speeding up the cycle.

If something is going wrong with sperm cell production, a man's bloodstream will often contain unusually high levels of FSH, since the pituitary keeps releasing more. A blood test to measure FSH levels is sometimes important in diagnosing the cause of infertility.

HOW MANY SPERM CELLS DO YOU NEED?

It is very difficult to tell an individual couple how many sperm are needed for conception. The old adage "It only takes one!" is true to the extent that if sperm and egg meet, fuse, and fertilize, a pregnancy can occur.

The average sperm count for men in the United States is about 60 to 70 million sperm per milliliter of semen, but these numbers are not required for a pregnancy to occur. According to the standards set by the World Health Organization (WHO), a sperm count of 20 million/ml or more is considered normal. Studies of large numbers of men who have fathered children and seek vasectomy for sterilization have shown that about 20 percent of these fertile men have sperm counts below the normal range.

Years ago, a study was done to try to find out how many sperm cells potentially reach an egg. Women about to have a hysterectomy underwent vaginal insemination just before surgery. One in 5,000 sperm cells placed in the vagina reached the cervical mucus—and only 1 out of 14 million reached the fallopian tube, where fertilization takes place. In a more recent, but similar, study, an average of 251 sperm cells were found in each fallopian tube 18 hours after vaginal insemination, suggesting a more optimistic ratio of sperm cells that almost make it to the finish line.

In the laboratory, when sperm cells are prepared for in vitro fertilization and put in a dish with a ripe egg, somewhere between 10,000 and 500,000 healthy sperm cells are needed to achieve good rates of fertilization. This seems quite a bit higher than the number of sperm cells that typically reach the egg from natural intercourse. It is not only the number of sperm cells that counts, however, but also their shape, called *morphology,* and their *motility,* or swimming power.

WHAT IS MOTILITY?

Motility is measured as the percentage of sperm cells that are moving when a semen analysis is done. Another factor is *forward progression,* or velocity, the ability of the sperm cells to swim ahead briskly. Sperm cells obviously need to be good swimmers to get from the vagina up to the fallopian tube to meet the egg. A combination of the number of sperm, their motility, and several other factors determines a man's potential for fertility. (See chapter 5 for an explanation of diagnostic tests for male infertility.)

THE MARATHON SWIM FOR THE EGG

Motility is so important because healthy sperm cells use their tails to swim forward through the female's reproductive maze in their search for the ripe egg. The first hurdle for the sperm cells is to swim through the *cervical mucus.* All during her menstrual cycle, a woman's cervix secretes a slippery fluid. As it collects on the walls of the vagina it acts as a natural cleansing system, removing bacteria and other particles as it flows out. At the time of ovulation, the cervical mucus becomes thinner and clearer to allow sperm cells to swim through its tiny channels much more easily. A woman may notice an increased, clear vaginal discharge several days before she would expect to be ovulating.

Once the sperm cells are past the cervix, it may only take a minute for some of them to cross the uterus and reach one of the two openings to the fallopian tubes. Researchers have used *sonograms* (images from sound waves) to discover that as a woman approaches ovulation, tiny uterine contractions become more frequent and can propel the sperm cells into the fallopian tubes. Even more interesting is that more of the sperm cells are directed into the tube that will receive the ripening egg.

FERTILIZATION: WHEN BOY MEETS GIRL

When the sperm cells reach the egg, their job is not yet done. Many reach this point, but only one sperm will cross the finish line. First the sperm must pass through the *cumulus* cells that surround the egg like little clouds. Then the sperm must bind to the shell, or *zona pellucida,* that surrounds the egg. At this time, the acrosomal cap, which covers most of the sperm head, releases some digestive chemicals to create a hole in the shell. This gets the sperm into the egg, in an outer area known as the *perivitelline space*. One sperm will fuse with the egg's membrane, preventing all others from entering. Then the head of the sperm dissolves, allowing the chromosomes from the egg and sperm to merge and the process of cell division to begin. The fertilized egg, or *zygote,* continues to travel slowly through the fallopian tube while it divides. When it reaches the uterine lining, if all goes well, it will implant and continue developing into an embryo.

DO SPERM CELLS COMPETE?

In a number of nonhuman species, it is well known that sperm cells from one male will attack and kill those of a second. In some animals, the semen of the first male to have intercourse with a female actually hardens into a vaginal plug, preventing sperm cells from another male from getting through the cervix.

A pair of researchers from England, Robin Baker and Mark Bellis, wrote a book suggesting that the sperm cells of human males also evolved to compete. They believe, based on studies of other primates such as chimpanzees, that in the course of human evolution, women typically would have intercourse with more than one man as part of a strategy to pick the father with the best genetic potential. Thus the males in a social group would compete with one another to sire children and have their genes live on.

Baker and Bellis theorize that only a small percentage of sperm cells are designed to run the marathon race to the egg. They call these "egg-getters." Other types of sperm, the "kamikazes" and "blockers," may have developed to seek out and kill sperm cells from another male. This theory is hard to prove, but leads to some interesting speculation. If sperm cells truly have different jobs, it may explain why even in men with normal fertility, the great majority of sperm cells do not have a perfectly normal shape. We will discuss ideas about human evolution and fertility more in chapter 18.

WHAT IS THE CHANCE OF A PREGNANCY?

Teenagers, or at least the parents of teenagers, all "know" that the chance of pregnancy is at least 90 percent if you have unprotected sex in the back seat of a car or if your condom leaks. When men or women discover an infertility problem, they often think with sad irony about all the years they spent worrying about contraception and unwanted pregnancy. In actuality, humans are not very fertile creatures, even in the best of circumstances.

A recent study of 200 healthy and presumably fertile couples trying to get pregnant monitored women's hormones carefully for the first signs of pregnancy. The couples were counseled on timing intercourse properly and followed for at least a year. The findings confirmed what researchers had previously suspected. The best pregnancy rates occurred during the first two cycles of trying. During these initial months, pregnancy rates were about 30 percent. Couples who did not get pregnant in the first two months had much lower rates of pregnancy per cycle.

Even the 30 percent pregnancy rates did not translate into 30 percent of women giving birth to a live baby, however. Of those very early pregnancies, almost a third ended in miscarriage, often before the woman even would have realized she was pregnant without the hormonal tests. About 1 in 5 couples did not conceive at all during the year of the study, which is similar to estimates that at least 15 percent of American couples will experience infertility.

When you are going through infertility treatment, you will have a more realistic idea of your chances of pregnancy if you compare the success rates of the treatments you are offered with these natural fertility rates. It is also helpful to have an idea of pregnancy rates in couples with infertility who do not receive treatment. In a study of over 2,000 couples with infertility who were followed for three years, a quarter experienced a live birth. For the couples who had a male factor in the infertility, however, the chance of having a baby was slightly less than half as good, so that about 1 out of 8 couples gave birth.

In this chapter we summarized the nuts and bolts of male fertility. Now we are ready to try to make some sense of the semen analysis and the other, even more specialized tests of sperm cell function that are used to diagnose a male fertility problem.

5

The Semen Analysis and Other Diagnostic Tests for Male Infertility

This chapter explains what is done in a semen analysis and the meaning of the various values in a laboratory report. We also describe other diagnostic tests that can be used to find the cause of abnormal semen quality. Ideally, three separate semen samples should be analyzed before drawing any final conclusions, since the quality of semen can vary quite a bit from one time to the next. If a man has had a recent high fever, a serious illness or an injury, or exposure to toxic chemicals, or has been taking medications that could affect his sperm production, the semen analysis may need to be delayed for about three months to allow the testicles to recover their normal function.

CHECKING OUT THE LABORATORY

The semen analysis is a very specialized test, and some laboratories are far more expert than others in performing it. How can you make sure that your semen analysis is done by a qualified laboratory? You can do a little research into the laboratory your doctor uses.

In some hospitals or clinics, semen analyses are rarely requested. Under these conditions the laboratory personnel, no matter how well trained and motivated, cannot perform the type of analysis your doctor will need to diagnose a male fertility problem. You should not hesitate to ask the laboratory director or technologist how often semen analyses are done and whether the laboratory employs technologists with specific training and experience in semen analysis.

Some laboratories use a special computerized machine, called a computer-assisted semen analyzer (CASA), to count sperm and measure their motion. Although laboratories that perform many semen analyses are more likely to have a CASA, the computerized analysis is not necessary for a high-quality semen analysis. The experience of the technologist is really the most important factor. A technologist can analyze semen quality using very simple instruments, as long as careful procedures are followed. In fact, a technologist may be more accurate than a computer in deciding which sperm are normal in shape (the morphology measure) and how rapidly they are moving.

Since 1992, all medical laboratories in the United States are required to have CLIA certification from the government. CLIA stands for the Clinical Laboratory Improvement Amendments of 1988, a set of regulations to ensure quality of laboratory services. These certificates are given at different levels for different types of labs. Many states also have their own requirements for laboratory certification. Technicians in a laboratory should be certified at their level of skill. You have a right to ask about the certifications of the laboratory and its personnel. You can ask your infertility specialist, or call the laboratory directly.

THE SEMEN ANALYSIS

One of the first things the technician does is to check whether the semen has *coagulated* or partially solidified. The semen coagulates right after ejaculation so that the sperm will be launched to the top of the vagina, around the cervix, rather than dripping down the vaginal walls. The semen then should begin to liquefy within the next 15 to 30 minutes. It is considered abnormal if semen is not completely liquefied within an hour. Liquefaction makes it easier for the sperm cells to swim out of the semen and through the woman's reproductive system. The viscosity, or texture, of the semen is rated on a scale from 0 (i.e., watery) to 4 (gel-like). A normal score is less than 3.

The *volume,* or amount, of the semen is also measured and should be 2.0 to 5.0 milliliters (5 milliliters is a teaspoon). A little more or less than these guidelines is not abnormal, however. The volume depends, in part, on how long it has been since a man's previous ejaculation when he gives the semen sample. To get the optimal volume, he should not ejaculate for two days before the day of the sample.

A very important measure is the *sperm concentration,* the actual number of sperm found in one milliliter of seminal fluid. It is also helpful to know how much fluid was in the total ejaculate—that is, the *semen volume.* Multiplying the two numbers together tells you how many sperm would be deposited in the vagina, ready to begin their journey to the *oocyte.* For example, if a man had a sperm concentration of 60 million per milliliter, and ejaculated 3.0 milliliters of semen, the total number of sperm he ejaculated would be 180 million. Officially, this total number is the *sperm count.* However, infertility specialists tend to use the terms "sperm concentration" and "sperm count" interchangeably. Whether the sperm count is performed with CASA or with a simple counting chamber matters little, as long as the technologist is experienced and accurate. Usually you will see the sperm "count" reported as the number of millions of sperm per milliliter of semen.

The sperm count or concentration can be confusing not only to patients but sometimes to their doctors. A low value would be less than 20 million sperm in each milliliter of fluid, or less than 40 million sperm in the entire ejaculate. Sometimes a man comes to our clinic having been told by his physician that his count is abnormally low. Yet he actually has a normal number of total sperm diluted in a larger than usual volume of semen. For example, if the laboratory said his sperm count was 15 million per milliliter (usually written as 15×10^6/ml), the count would seem slightly low. If the man's semen volume was a bit on the small side, let us say 1.5 ml, there would only be 22.5 million sperm in the ejaculate, which would indeed be abnormally low. On the other hand, if he ejaculated more semen than average—for example, 5.0 ml—he would have 75 million total sperm in his ejaculate, a number that would be considered adequate. Always ask about the sperm count and the semen volume to know if your values are in the normal range.

Once the semen has liquefied fully, the sperm motility, or percent and quality of moving sperm, can be measured. Ideally, more than 50 percent of the sperm cells should be vigorously motile. If a computerized analyzer is used, the actual sperm speed, the *velocity,* and the direction of movement can be measured. If these tests are performed by hand, the technologist first counts the number of moving sperm on a standard grid of squares placed under the microscope. The technician then rates the movement on a 4-point grading system, just like in school, with 4 given to the best, most active, forward-swimming sperm, and grade 1

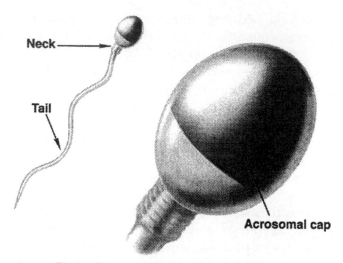

Neck

Tail

Acrosomal cap

Figure 5.1   A mature human sperm cell

used when the sperm are sluggish, just meandering around in one vicinity without moving off to find greener pastures. Using this method, we like to see a sperm motility of grade 3 or 4. If CASA is used to measure velocity, a speed of greater than 40 µ/second (microns per second) would be acceptable, but the faster the score, the better.

If a semen sample contains many nonmotile sperm—that is, sperm that are not moving at all—it does not necessarily mean that these sperm cells are dead. After all, a person sitting in one place may be very much alive. To see if a sperm is viable, a special stain is added to the sample after it is spread out on a microscope slide. The color changes tell the technologist if the sperm are dead or alive. We generally like to have more than 75 percent of the sperm be alive. Even in a normal sample, there are never 100 percent living sperm. Some cells are always dying, only to make way for newer, fresher sperm.

Another important aspect of the semen analysis is the morphology, the percent of sperm cells that have normal shapes. The sperm head should be oval in shape, with a smooth outline, and there are also special criteria for the size and shape of the acrosomal cap, the sperm neck, the midpiece, and the tail. At least 30 percent of sperm cells in the sample should be normal in shape. Although some computer programs try to analyze sperm shapes, an experienced technician currently does a more accurate job. Some laboratories use Kruger's Strict Criteria for Morphology, an even more precise rating system. The Kruger scoring should yield at least 14 percent normally shaped sperm cells. Men with

Kruger scores less than 4 percent may have poor fertilization using conventional in vitro fertilization (IVF).

TESTING FOR SIGNS
OF INFECTION OR INFLAMMATION

Semen samples should always be examined for signs that infection or inflammation could be present in the male's reproductive system. One such sign can be the presence of white blood cells in the semen. White blood cells (abbreviated as WBCs) are members of the body's response team to combat infections or inflammation.

A qualified laboratory will use special staining procedures to find out if there are an abnormal number of WBCs in the semen. It is especially important to use these stains if the tests show a lot of "round cells" in the semen, since immature sperm cells also may have a round appearance, making them easily confused with WBCs. In one common test, a stain called immunoperoxidase is used for this purpose. White blood cells are round, but so are immature sperm. Without proper laboratory tests, it is hard to tell one kind of cell from the other.

Not all laboratories perform these special tests for white cells. Unfortunately, men are sometimes diagnosed with an infection just on the basis of finding round cells in their semen. They may be treated with antibiotics for long periods of time because the round cells never go away—only to find out later that the cells were immature sperm, and not a sign of infection at all. Chapter 9 explains in detail the role of infection in male infertility. Sometimes the body's own immune system reacts to sperm cells as if they were foreign invaders that needed to be destroyed. The immune system then produces chemicals called antisperm antibodies. Tests for these chemicals are also described in chapter 9.

DIAGNOSTIC ALPHABET SOUP

Infertility specialists have invented some very tongue-twisting diagnostic labels for different types of male infertility. We mention them here because you may see them in your medical records or hear them discussed. Men with normal semen quality are called *normozoospermic* (or *normospermic)*. Men with low sperm concentrations are called *oligozoospermic*. If no sperm is seen in the semen, a man is *azoospermic*. A man with low sperm motility is *asthenozoospermic,* and a man with abnormally shaped sperm is *teratozoospermic.* When the semen analysis shows more than one problem, these labels are strung together, so that a man with low sperm concentration and motility, as well as abnormal morphology, would be *oligoasthenoteratozoospermic.* Say that three times in a row!

OTHER TESTS OF SPERM FUNCTION

Sperm cells not only have to survive the swim to the egg, but also must be able to fertilize it. Some tests of sperm cell function try to measure whether sperm cells would succeed in getting through the cervical mucus and then be capable of the act of fertilization. Such tests can be useful when the cause of male infertility is unclear, and when trying to make decisions such as whether to try intrauterine insemination, or to use conventional IVF, in which sperm cells are simply put in a dish with the oocyte in the lab, or to go directly to intracytoplasmic sperm injection (ICSI), in which a sperm cell is injected into each egg, bypassing the need for natural fertilization.

Some infertility specialists still use the *postcoital* test, in which a couple is asked to have intercourse at the time of ovulation and then come to the physician's office two to eight hours later. A sample of the mucus covering the woman's cervix is removed and examined to see whether it contains live sperm cells. The number of live sperm in each standard area, or field, of the microscope slide are counted and their motility is noted. This test tries to predict whether the sperm can transfer from the semen to the cervical mucus and then swim through. It also is used to see if the woman's mucus is thinning properly at ovulation. Otherwise it can be a barrier, rather than an aid, to conception. Abnormally thick mucus is sometimes called "hostile mucus."

Imagine how amorous you would feel if your wife woke you at five in the morning and said, "Honey, we have to have intercourse right away so that I can get to the gynecologist's office by eight! He's going to do a test to see how well your sperm can swim." Sometimes just getting in the mood for sex enough to get an erection is next to impossible. Some men also have later confessed to faking orgasm for the postcoital test (Yes, men can do this too!), because they simply could not reach a climax under that kind of pressure. In this situation, the wife may be devastated to learn that there were *no* sperm present in her mucus.

The postcoital test can be emotionally intrusive for a couple, and is only useful if the couple timed ovulation accurately and the man ejaculated normally during intercourse. Though a normal test can be valuable, the postcoital test is requested far less often today than in the past. One reason for skipping the postcoital test is that the ability of sperm to swim through cervical mucus can be tested in the laboratory without all that hassle. Cervical mucus from a cow can provide the Olympic swimming stadium for the sperm contestants. In the *bovine cervical mucus penetration assay,* some poor guy or gal (but luckily not you) has to collect the cervical mucus from cows at midcycle. This precious bodily substance is processed and placed into small, thin tubes. One end of the tube is open and placed into a very small cup containing your semen. Sperm swim into the mucus, hopefully racing toward the other end of the tube. After 90 minutes the technologist uses a microscope and a ruler to measure how far the sperm swam. Ideally, normal sperm swim over 30 millimeters in the time allotted—a gold medal performance for a tiny sperm.

There are no perfect laboratory tests to predict the ability of a man's sperm to fertilize an oocyte in real life. Fertilization is very complex, and depends not only on precise timing but on a series of chemical interactions between the sperm and egg. Even the most sophisticated laboratory cannot duplicate these conditions. The best that scientists can do is to try to simulate parts of the fertilization process. Dividing fertilization into steps, tests can be designed to try to identify potential problems. A number of these sperm function tests have been developed.

One of the first was termed the *zona-free hamster oocyte penetration assay,* or for short, the *sperm penetration assay* (SPA). Since it is the egg's shell, the zona pellucida, that accepts sperm from males of its own species, removing this barrier allows sperm to fuse with (but not fertilize) eggs of another species. This test shows whether a man's sperm are capable of this important fusion step in fertilization. Hamster eggs with their zona pellucida removed are put into an incubation dish with specially prepared human sperm cells. The number of sperm from the man being tested that penetrate the eggs is compared with the success of sperm from a human donor known to be fertile. Although real sperm and egg cells are used, they cannot develop into an embryo because humans and hamsters are too genetically different. Laboratories are not producing little "humsters." This test has also lost some of its popularity. It requires the availability of a small animal laboratory or the use of commercially sold frozen hamster eggs. Newer tests are being developed that may surpass the SPA in its ability to identify whether the sperm can attach and penetrate a human egg.

Since only human sperm have the ability to attach to and penetrate a human egg's zona pellucida, a test called the *hemizona assay* was developed. Human oocytes are needed for this test, and they are hard to obtain. Sources include unused eggs retrieved during IVF, eggs removed during an autopsy with permission from the family, or from ovaries removed in surgery. The eggs are cut in half under a microscope. One half of the shell, or zona pellucida, is incubated with the sperm cells of the man whose fertility is being tested. The other half is put in a container with sperm cells from a donor known to be fertile. The number of sperm cells that attach to the zona pellucida on each half (or hemizona) are counted and compared. Only the shell is used, so fertilization cannot take place and embryos do not develop. The results of this test have been used to predict fertilization in IVF. Because of the difficulties in obtaining human eggs, the hemizona assay is performed in very few laboratories, however.

Other tests of sperm-to-egg binding include the *acrosome reaction assay* and the *mannose binding assay.* These two tests are commonly performed together, although they take a good deal of labor. Under laboratory conditions designed to mimic those in the uterus and fallopian tubes, where fertilization will occur, the acrosome reaction test measures the percentage of sperm that release the chemicals from the acrosomal cap that aid in shell penetration. The mannose binding test identifies whether the sperm have enough of the chemical components needed in order to bind to the zona pellucida, making fertilization possible.

The *hypo-osmotic swelling test* is useful in identifying live sperm cells to use for ICSI when most cells in a sample have poor motility. When live sperm cells are put in a fluid less salty than their interior, they will absorb some of the fluid and swell. Dead sperm cells do not change in size.

HORMONE TESTS

Hormonal causes of infertility and their treatment are discussed in detail in chapter 11. For now, it is helpful to know that a blood test is often taken as part of an infertility workup to measure the hormones most important in male reproduction. The one most key to measure is follicle-stimulating hormone (FSH), which drives sperm production rates, as we saw in chapter 4. Tests are often run as well for luteinizing hormone (LH), prolactin, testosterone, and estradiol. If a man has any symptoms of an underactive or overactive thyroid, tests for thyroid hormones should also be done.

GETTING IMAGES OF
YOUR REPRODUCTIVE SYSTEM

Sometimes it is helpful to have a picture of your reproductive system, to make sure that all the parts are in working order. Simply taking an X ray will not work, since the X rays cannot create a clear enough picture of these soft tissues. One technique often used is to bounce sound waves off these organs to create images, using an ultrasound machine. The ultrasound device may be on a thin rod passed gently into your rectum or over the skin of your scrotum. The ultrasound is painless, and helps your doctor see your prostate, seminal vesicles, and ejaculatory ducts, or the testicle and its neighboring structures. Sometimes if a man has no sperm cells in his semen, and his seminal vesicles are enlarged, the ultrasound is used to guide a small needle through the rectum and into the seminal vesicles to aspirate (i.e., suck out) their contents.

If there is a suspicion that the sperm pathways are blocked, or obstructed, a special X ray of the vas deferens may be used. The *vasogram* is a surgical procedure performed in the operating room to identify whether there is an obstruction present in the vas deferens or ejaculatory ducts. It is usually performed at the time of corrective surgery. An incision is made in the skin of the scrotum, allowing the surgeon to pick up the vas deferens. Either a very small needle or a tiny catheter tube is placed into the inner channel, and a contrast liquid is injected. X rays are then taken of the sperm pathways. The contrast liquid that is injected into the vas deferens shows up as white on the X ray, and will not flow beyond any point of obstruction. A vasogram takes only a few minutes to perform, but is usually done as part of a corrective surgical procedure. A man can usually have this type of surgery as an outpatient, though some types of surgery require a brief hospital stay.

TESTICULAR BIOPSIES: OUCH!
ARE THEY AS BAD AS THEY SOUND?

If it is not possible to find live sperm cells in a man's semen, testicular biopsies may also be used to identify whether there is a problem with sperm cell production, if sperm production is normal but the transport pathways are blocked, or even to obtain sperm cells for IVF-ICSI. The very thought of someone cutting into such a sensitive part is enough to make the strongest man a bit queasy. In actuality, however, testicular biopsy is a relatively minor surgical procedure that should not result in a prolonged, painful period of healing. As with any surgery, there is always the risk of a complication, even with an expert and careful surgeon. The vast majority of men, however, have no problems. The experience of the surgeon in performing these biopsies can affect the likelihood of complications as well as the speed of a man's recovery.

Usually a testicular biopsy can be done in an outpatient surgery center, or even in an office setting, depending on the technique the surgeon uses. There are three methods used most commonly: fine needle aspiration, needle biopsy, and open testicular biopsy.

Fine needle aspiration is used when the physician primarily wants to know if there are mature sperm cells in the testis, or as a way to obtain sperm for IVF-ICSI. It is the most minor procedure, and has the advantages of being quick, inexpensive, and causing minimal pain. The drawback, however, is that it only gathers a tiny amount of tissue to examine, and so provides the least amount of information. The surgeon begins by cleansing the skin of the scrotum over the testicle and then numbing the area with a local anesthetic. The actual biopsy involves passing a thin hypodermic needle into the tissue of the testicle and drawing back on the attached syringe to aspirate some cells into the needle. The needle is withdrawn, and the material collected is placed on a glass slide, stained with colored dyes, and examined for sperm cells. The sperm may also be used for fertilization with IVF-ICSI.

Needle biopsy is different from needle aspiration because the biopsy needle itself is thicker and actually cuts out a small cylinder of testicular tissue. The needle used has a special, spring-loaded mechanism. A very sharp inner needle penetrates the testicle first, followed in the blink of an eye by a thin, outer sheath that actually shears off some tissue and stores it within a hollow area of the inner needle. The advantage is that a needle biopsy produces larger pieces of tissue to examine. At times, more than one sample needs to be taken. The discomfort is still minor, however, because a local anesthetic is injected beforehand to numb the area.

The *open biopsy* method is perhaps the oldest and probably still the most widely used way of obtaining tissue from the testicles. An open biopsy can either be done in an operating room or in an outpatient setting. Often, only a local anesthesia is needed, but a general anesthetic may be used, especially when a man has already had surgery on his testicle, or if his testicle is smaller or more sensitive than usual. If the only procedure needed is a biopsy, the surgeon makes an opening about a half inch long in the skin of the scrotum, allowing the surface of the testicle to be seen. The surgeon then makes a smaller opening in this surface, about a quarter inch long. A small amount of the tissue of the testicle pokes through the opening and is removed using a small and delicate pair of surgical scissors. This tissue is placed in a special solution to prepare it for staining and examination. It only takes a few sutures to close the small cut, and the patient usually goes home an hour or so later. The surgeon will typically ask the man to keep ice on the area of the incision on the first day, and not to do any vigorous activities for a few days. These instructions may vary from patient to patient, and from surgeon to surgeon, however.

The amount of pain during healing also varies quite a bit. One factor is how extensive the biopsy is. Sometimes a larger incision is used if the surgeon needs to explore and examine the entire contents of the scrotum. Occasionally more than one biopsy, or a larger sample of tissue, is needed. Another factor is a man's pain tolerance. Some men are quite sensitive to pain, whereas others have a higher pain threshold. Some men take narcotic pain medication after the biopsy and others use no pain medication at all.

Dr. Thomas recalls:

A number of years ago, I was invited to lecture and teach surgical techniques in a Middle Eastern country. I was introduced to a man whose brother I had treated successfully several years before for infertility. The second brother had a similar condition and needed a testicular biopsy. My former patient had already told his brother in sadistic detail how "painful" recovery from the biopsy had been, and had expressed doubt that the younger brother could handle it. I did operate on the second brother, and in fact his was the last procedure performed after a busy day of teaching and surgery. After I finished the biopsy, I changed my clothes to leave the hospital and go out to dinner. Waiting for us in the lobby was our host for the evening—the same man I had just biopsied an hour earlier! He had a smile on his face and was ready to eat! Sibling rivalry or a difference in pain threshold, who knows? Perhaps my skills had just improved over the years!

Now we turn our attention away from the laboratory and back to the real-life process of baby making. Although a number of couples reading this book may eventually conceive a child through fertilization taking place in a laboratory dish, most will succeed in getting the sperm to the egg the natural way, through sexual intercourse. The next chapter discusses how your sex life affects your fertility, and vice versa.

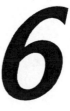

Starting the Production Line: Sex and Fertility

We have already discussed how sperm cells are manufactured and fertilization takes place. In most conceptions, sexual intercourse launches those sperm cells on their journey to find the egg. Problems in a couple's sex life can interfere with fertility if intercourse does not take place in an effective way at the right time. This chapter explains the basics of male sexual functioning and discusses the link between your sex life and your chances of conceiving.

WHAT CAUSES SEXUAL DESIRE?

Desire for sex is not so easy to define. It can include a mental longing for sexual contact, fantasies and pleasant genital feelings, or frustration at not having sex for a while. Sometimes desire seems to come out of the blue, but at other times (like when the calendar says it is ovulation time), drumming up a little passion can feel surprisingly like a chore. We know that certain areas of the brain play a role in sexual desire, but our map is very sketchy. The hormone testosterone, produced by the testicles, travels in the bloodstream to the brain where it acts to promote sexual desire. Men who have abnormally low levels of testosterone typically report losing their spontaneous interest in sex, although they may

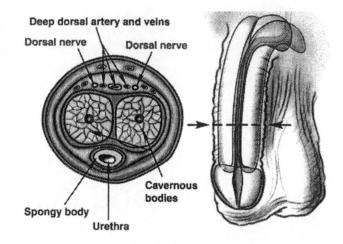

Figure 6.1   Diagram of the penis

be able to get turned on by trying lovemaking or watching an erotic video. Other chemicals in the brain that act as messengers between nerve cells also have an impact on desire for sex. One, called *dopamine,* probably helps increase desire. Another, serotonin, seems to block sexual desire.

Although a man's desire for sex typically leads to an erection, the two are not always linked. You can feel intense desire for sex without having a firm erection, and sometimes erections occur without any conscious sexual feelings (for example, when you wake up from sleep).

HOW ERECTIONS HAPPEN

To understand how erections work, you need to have an idea of what is inside the penis. As the illustration above shows, the shaft of the penis actually is made up of three chambers. Two sit side by side and make up the top half of the penis. They are called *cavernous bodies* and contain many tiny blood vessels lined by smooth muscle cells. When the nervous system sends a signal to the penis, the muscle cells relax, allowing blood to flow into the penis more rapidly. Spaces between the muscle cells fill up with blood, like a sponge soaking up water. As blood pressure inside the penis rises, the swelling tissue of the cavernous bodies presses against the small veins that normally drain blood from the penis. The veins are closed off, so that blood is trapped inside the cavernous bodies.

When the blood pressure rises to its maximum, the shaft of the penis becomes stiff.

The third chamber of the penis, the *spongy body,* runs along the bottom of the shaft and surrounds the urethra (the tube connecting the urinary bladder to the outside). It fans out to become the *glans,* or head of the penis. During erection, the glans also swells, but remains soft and spongy, providing a cushion for the vagina during intercourse.

Erotic messages from the brain carried by the nerves of the spinal cord trigger erections, but anxious thoughts can quickly deflate the penis. It was probably an advantage for early humans to be able to shut down sexual desire abruptly if danger loomed. You did not want to be smooching on the savanna, oblivious to the prowling saber-toothed tiger behind the tall grass. Perhaps as part of our sexual heritage, it is common for men to have trouble getting erections if they feel anxious and pressured to have intercourse at the right time of the month. Strategies to overcome these problems will be suggested in chapter 21.

As men age, medical problems that interfere with erections become more common. At around age 40, around 20 percent of men have moderate to severe difficulty with erections. By age 70, however, half of men have significant problems. Most are linked to unhealthy lifestyles or chronic illnesses that decrease the blood flow available to the penis. Not only are the arteries that bring blood to the penis rather small, but the soft tissue inside the cavernous bodies changes with aging or disease. It produces less *nitric oxide,* an important chemical that helps the tissue to relax during erection. Deposits of a substance called *collagen* can build up in the tissue, making it less soft and stretchy. To keep your penis youthful, follow the same advice that you would to keep a healthy heart: do not smoke; drink alcohol only in moderation; eat a diet low in fat; and exercise regularly. If an erection problem is keeping you from having intercourse, you can find information in chapter 21 about psychological or medical treatments that can enable you to function more normally.

THE MALE ORGASM: IT'S MORE COMPLICATED THAN IT FEELS

In chapter 4, we discussed how sperm cells and semen are made. During the male orgasm, all the ingredients of semen are combined with the ripe sperm cells that are stored in the vas deferens and the tail end of the epididymis. This mixing up occurs during the first stage of ejaculation, called *emission*. A man feels emission as the sensation of *ejaculatory inevitability*, better known as the point of no return. It is the pleasant feeling that a climax is about to happen. At that moment, the smooth muscle in the walls of the prostate gland and the seminal vesicles is contracting, squeezing out the fluid that makes up the semen. Ripe sperm cells travel up the two tubes of the vas deferens (refer back to the illustration on page 24) and mingle with the semen. A muscle between the prostate and the bladder shuts tightly and creates a pressure chamber, so the only path remaining for the semen is to travel outward, down the urethra. This sets the stage for the second stage of ejaculation—*expulsion*.

At the moment of ejaculation, the muscle between the prostate and the urethra opens, just as muscles at the base of the penis pump rhythmically, sending the semen out of the penis in spurts. The pleasure that goes with this physical process is the orgasm. Most of the sperm cells are in the first few spurts of semen. If ejaculation happens in a woman's vagina, the fastest sperm normally swim through her cervix within a few seconds.

WHAT IF A MAN CAN'T CLIMAX DURING INTERCOURSE?

Perhaps 5 percent of men have difficulty ejaculating in a woman's vagina. They typically can reach orgasm much more easily through their own self-touch, although a few men cannot have an orgasm at all except during their sleep. Over the years, some men will actually fake orgasm, so that their wives are not aware of the problem until the failure to conceive becomes an issue. If you have difficulty reaching orgasm during intercourse, treatments are available. Sex therapy techniques can sometimes help a man learn to reach orgasm inside the vagina (see chapter 21). Alternatively, an infertility specialist can use semen collected from masturbation or vibrator stimulation to inseminate the woman in the couple.

CAN YOU SPEED OR SLOW YOUR SPERM CELLS?

Couples who know they are up against a low sperm count or motility often hope they can do something special during lovemaking to increase their chances of pregnancy. There is no good scientific evidence that the position you use for intercourse affects your chance of conception. Advice to use the male-on-top position, or for the woman to lie on her back with her legs up for half an hour after intercourse, is just based on speculation. Probably the sperm cells that are going to have a chance at reaching the egg penetrate the cervix within the first couple of minutes after ejaculation. Keeping a pool of semen in the vagina, instead of letting it drip out after intercourse, is unlikely to increase your chance of pregnancy. Standing on your head is even more unnecessary! We suggest that you use the intercourse position that pleases you and helps you both to get in the mood at those crucial times.

Although some scientists thought that a woman's orgasm might help sperm cells get through the cervix by causing a kind of sucking action, this idea has not been confirmed. Again, there is no evidence that the woman's having an orgasm during intercourse, or even having simultaneous orgasms, will increase your odds of conception. Of course, there is also no evidence that it can hurt your chances.

There is one sexual practice that can interfere with sperm transport, however. If you want to become pregnant, *do not use a vaginal lubricant,* such as Vaseline, baby oil, or even K-Y Jelly, Astroglide, or Replens. A recent laboratory study found that even water-based lubricants stopped sperm cells almost as effectively as some contraceptive jellies that contain sperm-killing chemicals. The safest option is not to use any extra lubrication for intercourse. For most couples, spending extra time on caressing the woman during foreplay will increase her sexual arousal so that her natural lubrication will be all that is needed. If you cannot have comfortable intercourse without an extra lubricant, however, a small amount of saliva from either partner is probably the best choice.

TIMING INTERCOURSE
TO MAXIMIZE CONCEPTION

There is no question that intercourse needs to take place at the right time for a live sperm to meet a ripe egg. The window of opportunity for fertilization is fairly narrow. Recent studies agree that to have a chance of pregnancy, intercourse needs to occur during the five days that come before ovulation, or on the day of ovulation itself. Sperm cells may survive within a woman's body for more than 24 hours, but the ripe egg is available for less than a day. Sperm cells remain at the ready by lingering in small tunnels called *crypts* on the inner surface of the cervix. As the number of sperm cells around the upper vagina decreases, these stored sperm cells swim out to begin their journey in turn. A few sperm cells might survive for up to five days. The best chance of pregnancy (about 1 in 3 for a young couple with no fertility problem) is on the day of ovulation itself. Unfortunately, techniques many couples use to time intercourse to the right days of the cycle are of limited value, since they alert you that ovulation is already occurring. By then there is only one more highly effective day to have intercourse. This is true for basal body temperature charts and for the expensive kits that measure the surge of luteinizing hormone in the woman's urine. Not surprisingly, scientific studies have never proved that these methods increased couples' pregnancy rates.

We would advise a woman to keep track for a few months of the average length of her menstrual cycle, from first day of bleeding in one month to first day of bleeding in the next. Although the average cycle length is 28 days, cycles from 21 to 35 days are considered normal. Typically, the egg will be ripe about halfway through the average cycle. A week before this halfway point, start having intercourse on every other day, or every day if you have the energy! Continue this schedule until you are pretty sure the time of ovulation has passed.

For busy modern couples, having sex so often around midcycle can get stressful. You may find yourself trying to get in the mood for sex when all you really feel like doing is falling asleep, or setting the alarm to have a quickie before your morning shower. Business trips scheduled at the wrong time of the month become a marital crisis. When a woman has sex without much arousal, vaginal dryness often is a problem, especially since lubricants are not recommended when trying to conceive. Men suffer the anxiety of having to get erections or ejaculate on demand, sometimes leading to sexual problems that only occur when the pressure is on at midcycle. Chapter 21 suggests some tactics to overcome these performance anxieties.

As an experienced sex therapist, Dr. Schover recommends intercourse every other day the week before and during ovulation—the minimum schedule of sexual intercourse likely to be efficient for conception. Dr. Thomas, however, often suggests that couples have daily intercourse and sometimes tells them to have intercourse at least every other day all month! Although Dr. Schover wonders if this difference reflects their ethnic backgrounds (she calls her schedule the Jewish American Princess's path to pregnancy), or a female versus male strategy, Dr. Thomas may have some science on his side. (He also has four children to Dr. Schover's one.) A study from Israel (so much for ethnicity) published in 1994 compared semen analyses spaced just 24 hours apart in a large group of men with normal fertility, and in another big group of men with poor sperm counts and/or motility. Although sperm counts in the second daily sample decreased significantly in the men with normal fertility, sperm counts actually increased in the men with poorest fertility, and remained stable in those with more moderate fertility problems. The authors concluded that men with low sperm counts or motility could increase their chances of a pregnancy by having intercourse at least once, if not twice, a day! Perhaps you are one of the rare, but lucky, couples who enjoy daily sex. If so, great! If not, you will need to find your own balance between your longing for a child and your ability to get in the mood for sex.

KEEPING SPERM CELLS FRESH

Even if you are going through assisted reproduction procedures like intrauterine insemination (IUI) or in vitro fertilization (IVF) that do not involve having intercourse to get pregnant, a man should try to ejaculate regularly, especially as it gets close to the time that he will need to provide a semen sample. You only need to abstain for a couple of days before a sample, unless your doctor instructs otherwise. Ejaculation at other times can take place during intercourse, or from other types of sexual stimulation that you find comfortable. No matter how you reach an orgasm, ejaculating a couple of times a week ensures that the sperm cells will be as freshly minted and healthy as possible.

WHEN INTERCOURSE
IS JUST NOT ENOUGH

Although physicians have been surprised by couples who conceive a "miracle baby" despite the husband's very abnormal semen analysis, more typically there are some couples who are unable to get pregnant through sexual intercourse. Not only sperm count and motility, but the concentration of motile sperm cells in the semen, predict how long it may take a couple to become pregnant. When problems are severe, the only realistic hope may be to use assisted reproductive technology, such as intrauterine insemination or in vitro fertilization (see chapter 16).

Part One of this book has looked at the impact of a diagnosis of male infertility and given you an idea of how to find expert help, how to understand the process of reproduction and the diagnostic tests for problems on the male side, and how your sex life can contribute to fertility problems. Next, in Part Two, we explain the medical causes of male infertility as well as the treatments that may help overcome these problems.

Part Two
Understanding Male Infertility: Causes and Treatments

7

Holes in Our Genes:
Inherited Causes
of Infertility

How often does male infertility have a genetic cause? More often than anyone suspected until recently. In chapter 4 we explained how sperm and egg transmit the father's and mother's genes to their offspring. Sperm cell production itself is controlled by a number of different genes. When these genes mutate (i.e., the genetic code develops a spelling mistake), infertility can result.

Men normally have two sex chromosomes, an X and a Y, whereas women have two Xs. The Y chromosome is a very special one. It is the only chromosome that does not pair up completely with its mate during cell division. Y's partial stand-alone nature may have allowed its genes to mutate faster than those on other chromosomes. As a result, the human Y chromosome has developed some altered genes that enable men to be superb sperm producers. On the downside, these changes also leave the genes on the Y chromosome more vulnerable to mistakes that could interfere with fertility.

Damaged genes on the Y chromosome are not the only genetic cause of male infertility. A variety of other inherited problems can affect sperm production, including several genetic diseases. Someday medicine may be able to correct these problems with gene therapy. In the meantime, new treatments like in vitro fertilization (IVF) with intracy-toplasmic sperm injection (ICSI) enable men with very low sperm counts to father sons who may grow up to have the same sperm-production problem as Dad. Although most genetic problems have no cure yet, it is important to understand them and their impact on you and your potential children.

DO YOU HAVE AN EXTRA X?

About 1 in 500 men are born with an extra X chromosome, so that each cell contains two Xs and a Y. This is called *Klinefelter syndrome,* named after a physician who first described it early in the 20th century. Men with this syndrome are tall on the average, and have long arms and legs. Some may have specific learning problems, though their overall intelli-gence is usually normal. Their testicles are small and firm, but these men typically have normal sex lives. About a third of men with the syn-drome develop some breast enlargement at puberty, which sometimes leads to the diagnosis of the condition.

The changes in a man's appearance or well-being are subtle, howev-er, and a number of men do not find out they have an extra X until they discover they are infertile. Klinefelter syndrome is found in about 11 percent of men who have no sperm cells in their semen, and 2 percent of men with low sperm counts. Some men with Klinefelter syndrome who have no sperm cells in their semen do have very small islands of tis-sue in the testicles where sperm are being produced. About 15 percent of men with Klinefelter have a *mosaic* condition, however. This is a genetic term that means some of the cells in their body are XXY, and some are normal XY cells. Men with mosaicism often do not have the typical features of Klinefelter syndrome, and may produce more sperm cells. Some men with complete Klinefelter syndrome have fathered chil-dren recently through IVF-ICSI using cells retrieved by biopsying their testicles.

Whether a man has a complete or a mosaic form of Klinefelter syn-drome, he may produce sperm cells that contain both an X and a Y chromosome. There is a chance that his son conceived through ICSI could also have Klinefelter syndrome. As we discuss later in this chap-ter, it may be possible to use some new techniques called *preimplanta-tion genetic diagnosis* with IVF to identify embryos with a normal num-ber of X and Y chromosomes for uterine transfer.

The diagnosis of Klinefelter syndrome may come as an emotional shock. Some men question whether they are "truly male" if they have an extra X chromosome. Manhood is not only a biological fact, defined by having a penis, testicles, and making the hormone testosterone; it also is a psychological state. Men with Klinefelter syndrome are no less masculine than any other men. Chromosomes are only one part of the picture when it comes to gender. The extra X chromosome that creates the condition may come either from a man's father or his mother. On the average, Klinefelter syndrome occurs more commonly when parents are older.

DO YOU HAVE AN EXTRA Y?

Another error, which occurs in about 1 in 1,000 male babies, is being born with an extra Y chromosome. Most of these men have normal fertility, but occasionally the extra Y interferes with sperm cell production. Just as XXY men are not feminine, XYY men do not seem to be supermasculine. In the past, research suggested that XYY men might be more likely to commit violent crimes, but this theory did not hold up. Men with XYY are taller than average, and often have some problems with specific types of learning skills.

IS YOUR Y MISSING SOMETHING?

At least three areas of the Y chromosome contain genes important to sperm cell production. Sometimes the Y loses a tiny piece of its genetic material, interrupting the genetic code. This is called a *microdeletion*. In men who have severe male infertility—that is, they either have no sperm cells in their semen or have very low sperm counts (below 2 million per ml)—somewhere around 9 percent to 18 percent are found to have microdeletions on the Y chromosome, showing that their infertility has a genetic basis. Since a son gets his Y chromosome from his father, male babies conceived through IVF-ICSI will also be born with the same microdeletion as the father had and will also have fertility problems as adults, although they should be healthy in all other ways. As the genes on the Y chromosome are mapped fully, genetic tests will be available for even smaller mutations that may affect fertility but cannot be found with our current techniques.

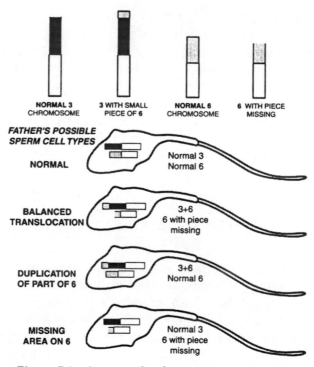

Figure 7.1   An example of a genetic translocation

TRANSLOCATIONS:
WHEN GENES GET CONFUSED

When an embryo is first developing, the chromosomes sometimes get shuffled incorrectly. A piece of genetic material from one chromosome—for example, in pair number 3—gets attached to another one—for example, in pair number 6—by mistake. This is called a *balanced translocation*. As the embryo grows into an infant, the cells in its body contain all the genes necessary for life, but a few are rearranged. When a man with a translocation makes sperm cells, some will contain only the normal chromosomes, but others will have an extra section of genes or will be missing some genetic material (see Fig. 7.1). If abnormal sperm cells fertilize an egg, the most common outcome is that the embryo fails to develop, and an early miscarriage results. Sometimes, however, a baby will be born with birth defects.

An even more common type of gene interchange is called a *Robertsonian translocation*. The shorter halves of two different, unpaired chromosomes get lost during cell division, and the longer halves of the two chromosomes fuse together. Although some genes are lost, they are very minor ones and the person with the translocation is healthy and appears totally normal. Again, however, that person's offspring may end up with a more serious problem because they have missing genes or extra ones.

In general, the rate of translocations in men is about 1 in 500. In men with very low sperm counts, however, the rate is at least 2 in 100, and may be higher in men with no sperm cells in their semen (and no obstruction of the sperm pathways). Translocations can be diagnosed by a test called *karyotyping,* described in detail later in this chapter. Blood cells are cultured and a picture is made of the chromosomes so that their number and shape can be checked. If a man has a translocation, genetic counseling can help the couple understand the potential outcomes if they try for a pregnancy. If they decide to go ahead with infertility treatment, prenatal diagnosis or, in some centers, preimplantation, genetic diagnosis can be done to detect potential birth defects. These techniques also bring ethical dilemmas, as couples may be asked to decide whether they want to terminate a pregnancy or destroy an embryo, as we discuss later in this chapter.

CONGENITAL BILATERAL ABSENCE
OF THE VAS DEFERENS (CBAVD)

When a man's semen sample turns out to have no sperm cells in it, there is about a 2 percent chance that the problem is *congenital bilateral absence of the vas deferens* (CBAVD). As we discussed in chapter 4, the vas deferens is the pair of tubes that transport mature sperm cells from the epididymis to the area where semen is mixed together. Without these tubes, sperm cells are all dressed up with nowhere to go. Men with CBAVD will often have a low volume of fluid at ejaculation because their seminal vesicles are not well developed. Other tip-offs to this condition include a low level or absence of fructose in the seminal fluid, and failure of the semen to coagulate after ejaculation.

In recent years scientists discovered that about two-thirds of men with CBAVD have mutations in the gene associated with *cystic fibrosis.* Cystic fibrosis is one of the most common genetic illnesses in Caucasians. A baby is born with cystic fibrosis if both parents contribute a mutated copy of the *cystic fibrosis transmembrane receptor* (CFTR) gene on chromosome number 7. About 1 in 25 whites of European ancestry carries this mutation, meaning that they have one good copy of the gene and one with a spelling mistake. A person who carries only one bad copy of the gene does *not* have cystic fibrosis, but is a *carrier.* When both parents are carriers of a CFTR mutation, they have a 1 in 4 chance of having a baby with cystic fibrosis.

About 1 in 2,500 Caucasian babies is born with this disease. Its symptoms include thick mucus that clogs up the lungs, creating a risk for bacterial infections which can lead to early death from lung failure. Another problem is that the pancreas cannot produce the correct juices to aid digestion, so that children with cystic fibrosis are malnourished. Medication is now available to replace the missing pancreas enzyme, and with special therapy for their lungs, the average life span for people with cystic fibrosis is now about 40 years. The great majority of men with cystic fibrosis have no vas deferens, and thus have no sperm cells in their semen. Since people with cystic fibrosis are now living longer, however, some are interested in having children of their own.

A particular mutation in the CFTR gene, called Delta-F508, is responsible for about 70 percent of the spelling errors in this gene. Up to 600 other mutations in the CFTR gene have also been found, however. Some produce more severe health problems than others, so a child's health may vary, depending on which mutations have led to the disease.

Men who have one normal CFTR gene and one copy with a Delta-F508 mutation are often born without a vas deferens, even though they have normal lungs and digestion. A number of other combinations of mutations can also lead to CBAVD without causing cystic fibrosis. Some men with CBAVD actually have two mildly damaged copies of the CFTR gene, but do not have the other symptoms of the disease. Some men with only one vas deferens tube also have CFTR mutations. To complicate things a little more, some men with a CFTR gene mutation have both tubes of the vas deferens, but have poor sperm counts. The CFTR gene may have some influence on sperm production itself.

Until the use of IVF with ICSI, men with cystic fibrosis or with CBAVD could not father children. Now we can retrieve sperm cells directly from a man's epididymis or testicle and use them in the laboratory for IVF with ICSI. Will this lead to more babies born with cystic fibrosis? Luckily, sophisticated genetic tests are available that can find mutations on the CFTR gene using cells from a simple blood test. Good commercial laboratory tests for the CFTR gene screen for the most common 30 to 70 mutations. For men with CBAVD, it also may be helpful to include a special test for the *intron 8 splice 5T variant,* a variation in the

CFTR gene that is not classified as a mutation, but does contribute to about half of CBAVD cases.

A man with CBAVD should have cystic fibrosis gene testing, so that he knows his exact genetic situation. If he has a CFTR gene mutation, his wife should also be tested. If she has two unaltered copies of the gene, it is highly unlikely that their child will have cystic fibrosis. If the baby is a boy, however, there is a chance he will have CBAVD, just like his father. The chance of CBAVD in a son is difficult to predict, since the CFTR gene interacts with other, unknown genes to produce the syndrome. It could be as high as 1 out of 2 for some couples, and far lower for others. Most couples faced with this problem decide to go ahead with infertility treatment, since they feel that infertility in a male is treatable, and not a major barrier to a good quality of life for their potential child. Some choose not to have a child, however, or to use a sperm donor to avoid the risk of infertility in a son.

There is also a small chance, estimated at 1 in 800, that a baby could be born with cystic fibrosis, even if both the mother's and father's gene test comes out normal. This uncertainty happens because labs do not test for all the hundreds of known mutations in the gene. Such a test would be extremely expensive.

One recent study found a fourfold increase in CFTR gene mutations in a group of men with very low or absent sperm counts, but without known CBAVD. A more careful examination of a group of men about to try IVF-ICSI did not find any unusual rates of CFTR gene mutations, however. Some experts recommend CFTR gene testing for all men with unusually low sperm counts, but others only routinely recommend it for men who have an absent vas deferens. In 1997, the National Institutes of Health suggested that testing for the CFTR gene be offered to all Caucasian couples of European descent as part of planning for a healthy pregnancy.

OTHER GENETIC CAUSES
OF MALE INFERTILITY

At least one known inherited abnormality, called the *immotile cilia syndrome,* is known to damage sperm motility. Although the gene that causes this problem has not yet been located, a mutation occurs in about 1 out of 20,000 men. Along with sperm that do not move their tails, these men typically have had sinus problems since early childhood and a chronic cough. One of the more severe variations of this disorder, called Kartagener syndrome, is inherited in an *autosomal recessive* pattern. Autosomal means that it is not related to the X or Y chromosomes, but to one of the other 22 chromosome pairs. Recessive means that as with cystic fibrosis, you only have the syndrome if each of your parents carries one abnormal copy of the gene, which they each pass on to you. You then have two mutated copies of the gene. Since a person who carries only one altered copy of the gene would not have the physical symptoms of immotile cilia syndrome, your parents could be completely healthy and fertile.

Male infertility can also occur when an inherited genetic change affects the way that male hormones are produced or used by the body. Male infertility is also common in some blood disorders, such as sickle-cell anemia or beta thalassemia, and some types of muscular dystrophy. If a man with infertility has a family history of the same problem, or if men in the family develop neurological disease (muscle weakness, trouble speaking and swallowing) in their adult years, it may be helpful to have formal genetic counseling.

WHO SHOULD CONSIDER
HAVING GENETIC COUNSELING?

As scientists continue to map out the genes that make up the blueprint of a human, more genetic counseling and testing will be available. Already, in programs that offer IVF with ICSI, genetic testing is showing that about 4 percent of men have abnormal karyotypes and about 9 percent have microdeletions of the Y chromosome. About 1 in 100 babies born from ICSI have an abnormal number of sex chromosomes, compared to 1 or 2 in 1,000 babies in the general population. Many IVF-ICSI programs, especially those in Europe, where genetic testing is covered under national health insurance plans, request or require that all couples have genetic counseling and testing beforehand.

Of course, there are some men who are using IVF-ICSI because of a past vasectomy or an obstruction of the sperm pathways related to a past infection. The likelihood that they have a genetic problem related to their infertility is small.

In the United States, where genetic testing is expensive and not always covered by private insurers, the standards for offering genetic counseling vary, but there is a growing trend to suggest it to all couples contemplating IVF-ICSI. Men with CBAVD should definitely be offered genetic counseling and testing for the CFTR gene. Some programs suggest genetic counseling for all couples in which the male partner has a sperm concentration of less than 10 million per ml. Other programs use a 2 million per ml criterion, or only suggest genetic counseling for men whose sperm cells need to be retrieved from the testicle.

Ultimately, you may need to decide for yourselves how important you consider genetic counseling, genetic testing, and prenatal testing. The next sections of this chapter should help you make a more informed choice.

WHAT IS GENETIC COUNSELING?

Genetic counseling involves professionals trained in medical genetics meeting with you to take a family history that assesses your risk to have or to pass on a genetic problem, to educate you about the problem in question, and to discuss the options you have for genetic or prenatal testing. Ideally, genetic testing should not be done until you have had genetic counseling. Genetic counseling is usually performed by a certified *genetic counselor.* Genetic counselors have at least two years of course work beyond a four-year college degree. They also have supervised training in interacting with patients, and over a period of several years must pass an examination by the American Board of Genetics Counselors to be certified. Genetic counselors try to give you a clear understanding of your risks and options, without directing you into one particular path. During the course of genetic counseling you may also meet with a *medical geneticist,* a physician who has completed a special fellowship program and is board certified in this specialty.

GENETIC TESTS FOR MEN WITH INFERTILITY

We will describe the genetic tests currently available for men with infertility, but this field is changing so rapidly that new developments may already have occurred before this book could be published.

The Karyotype. A karyotype usually just involves getting a routine blood sample. The blood cells are then cultured for two or three days and treated with chemicals that allow a picture to be made of the 23 pairs of chromosomes. The number and the shape of the chromosomes are examined carefully for abnormalities. A normal male karyotype is called 46, XY; that is, it has 44 regular chromosomes, plus one X and one Y. A normal female karyotype would be 46, XX. Karyotypes can diagnose syndromes in which a man has the wrong number of X or Y chromosomes, or has a chromosome translocation. It also can identify problems such as Down syndrome, in which there are three number 21 chromosomes instead of two.

Microdeletions of the Y Chromosome. Genetic tests to find tiny missing segments of DNA on the Y chromosome are still mainly performed in research laboratories. If you feel that having a microdeletion might change your choices about having a child, your infertility specialist may be able to send a sample of your blood to a laboratory with special expertise in these tests. The laboratory will use sophisticated tests to check the completeness of the chromosome in the areas important for sperm production.

Although Y microdeletions have no known health impact except on sperm cell production, they will be passed on from father to son if IVF-ICSI is successful. A few couples might decide they did not want to have a male child who would inherit the father's infertility. Their options would be to use preimplantation genetic diagnosis or prenatal diagnosis to prevent the birth of a son, to decide not to have children, to use sperm from a donor, or to adopt.

TESTING FOR THE
CYSTIC FIBROSIS GENE

Although the genetic test for cystic fibrosis mutations is most strongly indicated for couples in which the man has CBAVD, it is recommended by the National Institutes of Health (but not so far by the American College of Gynecologists) for any couple of Caucasian ancestry planning a pregnancy. The test looks for actual patterns in the DNA that makes up the gene. A genetic counselor can use the test results to predict a couple's risk of having a baby with cystic fibrosis. It may also be possible to estimate the risk of having a son with CBAVD, although the genetics of this condition are so complex that accurate predictions are not always possible. The couple can use their risk estimates to decide whether to pursue prenatal testing or preimplantation genetic diagnosis.

PRENATAL DIAGNOSTIC TESTING

Prenatal diagnostic testing allows physicians to look for genetic abnormalities or birth defects in the fetus during pregnancy. A variety of techniques are available.

Ultrasonography. A picture of the fetus can be made, using sound waves. Ultrasonography does not involve the risk of radiation to the fetus that an X ray would. During the first 13 weeks of pregnancy, an ultrasound may be used to show that the fetus has a heartbeat, is the expected size given the date the couple believes conception took place (or the date of embryo transfer if the pregnancy resulted from IVF), and that the fetus is located properly inside the uterus. Around week 16 to 18 of the pregnancy, a more detailed ultrasound scan can be performed. A skilled ultrasonographer can find problems with the fetal heart, the kidneys, the brain, the spine, or other organs, although no ultrasound is 100 percent accurate. An abnormal scan might also indicate a genetic problem. The ultrasound image is also necessary to guide other diagnostic tests, such as amniocentesis or chorionic villus sampling (CVS).

The Triple Screen. Another very routine way of spotting a problem is called the *triple screen*. A blood sample is taken from the mother at around week 15 of pregnancy. The levels of three hormones are tested: alpha-fetoprotein, unconjugated estriol, and human chorionic gonadotropin. If the test is abnormal, the fetus may have Down syndrome or a *neural tube defect* (i.e., a problem, such as spina bifida or anencephaly, in which the brain or spinal cord is not developing properly). This test misses about 30 percent to 40 percent of Down syndrome cases, so it is not as accurate as the more complicated tests we will discuss later. Because this test is designed for screening, the rate of false positive results is high; that is, the test is abnormal but the fetus is, in fact, healthy. An abnormal result is usually followed up with a detailed ultrasound or an amniocentesis.

Amniocentesis. Some readers may be familiar with the procedure called *amniocentesis*. Between weeks 15 and 18 of pregnancy, an ultrasound image is used to guide a needle through the mother's belly and uterine wall into the amniotic fluid that surrounds the fetus. The amniotic fluid contains living cells shed by the fetus. These cells are grown in culture and then used for genetic testing. The most common test performed is a karyotype of the fetus, which is usually available in 10 to 14 days. Most other genetic tests that can be done on an adult can also be performed on the fetal cells, however, including tests for cystic fibrosis or other genetic diseases in which the specific gene mutation is known. The accuracy of a chromosome test from amniocentesis is about 99 percent. An amniocentesis increases the risk of miscarriage by about one-half of a percent, or one chance in 200.

Chorionic Villus Sampling (CVS). Amniocentesis is performed fairly late in a pregnancy. If a couple were to decide to terminate a pregnancy at this time, it could be a complicated and traumatic procedure. *Chorionic villus sampling* is done at weeks 10 to 12, and involves using a thin plastic catheter to gather a small sample of the placental tissue, which shares the same genetic makeup as the fetus. The catheter is guided by ultrasound through the mother's cervix (although occasionally the test is done like an amniocentesis, with a needle through her abdomen). The tissue is cultured and results are usually available more quickly than for amniocentesis. The risks of miscarriage from the procedure are a bit higher, 1 percent to 2 percent. Again, the accuracy is about 99 percent. The advantage is having knowledge about the health of the fetus earlier in the pregnancy, both for reassurance and for decision making.

Percutaneous Umbilical Blood Sampling (PUBS). Although it is rare, sometimes genetic testing requires an actual sample of blood from the fetus. Sometimes this is necessary if the results of the amniocentesis or CVS indicate mosaicism (i.e., some cells appear to have normal chromosomes but other cells were abnormal). At weeks 16 to 20 of pregnancy, ultrasound guidance can be used to actually put a needle into the umbilical cord and draw a sample of fetal blood.

Preimplantation Genetic Diagnosis. Perhaps the most amazing form of prenatal diagnosis is the use of genetic testing to choose healthy embryos to transfer in IVF. When an embryo reaches 8 to 16 cells in size, one of the cells can be removed without apparent damage to the potential of the embryo to keep on growing. That cell can be cultured, and its genetic material used for genetic testing. To test for a few genetic diseases, such as Tay-Sachs disease, muscular dystrophy, or *Huntington's disease* (a deadly disease that usually begins in middle age and involves deterioration of the central nervous system), the embryo may need to be grown for another two days to the *blastocyst* stage, so that several cells can be removed. Couples are given the choice to transfer only the embryos free of the genetic problem to the mother's uterus and to decide the fate of the other embryos.

If the goal is to transfer fresh embryos, the genetic testing needs to use techniques that will find a mutation very rapidly. Sometimes the embryos could be frozen while testing proceeded and then transferred in a later cycle, but the chance of a pregnancy would be lessened.

Preimplantation genetic diagnosis is still a very new procedure, and only available in a few centers around the United States. It has been used to choose female embryos to avoid transmitting a genetic disease that is sex-linked (for example, diseases like hemophilia that only occur in males). Some of these diseases are well known, but a specific gene has not yet been identified for testing. It has also been used to choose embryos that do not carry genes for specific disorders, such as cystic fibrosis or Tay-Sachs disease. It can be used to choose potentially healthy embryos when one parent has a genetic translocation. Although no obvious health consequences of preimplantation genetic diagnosis have been seen in the children born, it is still a new procedure.

Preimplantation genetic diagnosis will be available for more and more genetic problems in the next few years, but it will remain a very difficult and expensive way to have a healthy child. Couples who would not normally need to resort to IVF to have a baby will have to undergo the medical and financial risks of an IVF cycle. The genetic testing also adds considerable cost, which may or may not be covered by insurance.

Eliminating embryos that carry genetic mutations for a disease may not leave many healthy embryos for transfer, decreasing the chance of a pregnancy. Nature also makes many genetic mistakes in embryos, which probably accounts for some of the limited success in IVF. Most often, severe genetic problems in an embryo simply lead to a failure to implant or an early miscarriage. In a recent study, a genetic analysis was made of leftover embryos from cycles of IVF. Less than half of the embryos were normal on all the genetic tests used (although remember that these were the embryos not chosen for transfer to the mother).

Concerns have been raised that preimplantation genetic diagnosis will be used by some couples to select desired genetic traits in a child. For example, preimplantation genetic diagnosis can already select embryos with normal XX or XY sex chromosomes, allowing couples to choose the gender of their child. In the future, when more genes have been identified, it could perhaps be used by affluent couples who want a child who will be smarter or more athletic. Most physicians and bioethicists reject the idea of using preimplantation genetic diagnosis (or even new, less-invasive laboratory techniques that use tiny differences in weight to sort X versus Y chromosome–bearing sperm for use in intra-uterine insemination, or IUI) simply to choose the gender of a child. There is also some controversy over whether to use preimplantation genetic diagnosis only to prevent diseases that affect children, like cystic fibrosis, or to test for diseases that show themselves later in life, such as Huntington's disease or inherited breast cancer.

Of course, using preimplantation genetic diagnosis also implies that a couple is willing to leave some embryos unused if they carry an abnormality. A number of couples may find this unacceptable, from an ethical or religious standpoint. New technologies bring new dilemmas.

Who Uses Prenatal Diagnosis? Many couples have prenatal diagnosis for reassurance, since in the great majority of cases the tests show that the fetus is developing normally. Other couples use prenatal diagnosis because they want to be emotionally prepared for the birth of a child with a medical problem. In the near future, prenatal diagnosis may allow physicians to intervene to correct potential diseases with prenatal surgery or gene therapy. Some couples also choose to have testing because they would consider terminating a pregnancy in the event of a severe birth defect or genetic disease.

We recently interviewed all of our IVF couples about their intentions to use prenatal diagnosis if they had a pregnancy. Many of those who had male factor infertility were not interested in having genetic counseling or prenatal diagnostic testing. Couples having IVF-ICSI were not very concerned about the idea of transmitting the problem of male infertility to a son. They believed that similar or superior infertility treatments would be available in the future for their children. Even when couples were told about the small risk of a severe birth defect related to a balanced translocation, they sometimes refused karyotyping because it would add several hundred dollars to the cost of their treatment. If the man had CBAVD, all couples had cystic fibrosis gene testing, however.

Couples who have conceived a pregnancy through the tedious process of IVF may also be more concerned than most about the slight risk of miscarriage after amniocentesis or CVS. On the other hand, couples who have already had a child born with a genetic disease, or have seen its ravages in nieces and nephews, may be more motivated to use prenatal diagnosis. Even within these groups, many want the information to prepare themselves emotionally for having an affected child, rather than to make a choice about pregnancy termination. Couples may choose termination if they feel the burden of a disease would be severe enough to destroy a child's quality of life or to be a tragedy for the family. Religious or moral values about pregnancy termination or the fate of embryos also play an important role in these choices. Other options to avoid transmitting a genetic disease include using a donated sperm or oocyte to conceive, or adopting a child. These will be discussed in Part Three.

THE HEALTH OF
CHILDREN BORN FROM IVF-ICSI

Using IVF-ICSI to bypass fertilization does not appear to create genetic flaws in itself as a technique. As we have seen in this chapter, however, men who need to use IVF-ICSI to have a child may have a higher than usual risk of passing on a genetic problem. Genetic studies of babies born from IVF-ICSI have mostly been reassuring, in that rates of major birth defects were no different than those in babies conceived by conventional IVF or from natural intercourse (the expected rate of birth defects is between 2 and 5 percent). As we mentioned before, with IVF-ICSI, there has been a slight increase of babies born with an abnormal number of sex chromosomes, however (1 in 100 instead of the usual 1 or 2 in 1,000 newborns). A comparison of births from pregnancies conceived with sperm cells that were ejaculated, sperm cells taken from the epididymis, and those found directly in testicular tissue did not find any major differences in the outcomes of the pregnancies. As with pregnancies from regular IVF, rates of multiple pregnancies were higher than usual, resulting in more premature and low-birth-weight babies.

Recently, two fairly large series of children born from IVF-ICSI were examined. In an infertility program in Australia, about 15 percent of male toddlers born from ICSI had developmental test results that could signal learning problems when they become of school age. Similar testing of children in Belgium, however, found no unusual problems in an ICSI group. In fact, the children were unusually advanced for their ages. Although the Australian study suggests that a subset of these children may have problems, the test they used was developed for American children and may not have had accurate results in Australia. These test scores also are not very strong predictors of later performance in school.

The best guarantee of having healthy children for couples who need to use IVF-ICSI is to use genetic counseling and testing to identify genetic risk factors, and if possible, reduce the chance of transmitting them.

In this chapter we examined the way in which our very genes can shape male fertility. In the next chapter we move from the level of the laboratory and microscope to problems that can be spotted with the naked eye. We will talk about infertility related to problems in the formation of the male reproductive organs—for example, testicles that do not descend into the scrotum or a urinary opening on the wrong spot on the penis.

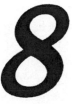

Developmental Problems That Cause Infertility

During the weeks that a fetus is growing, parts of the male reproductive system occasionally fail to develop correctly. This chapter discusses some developmental problems that can interfere with a man's fertility.

WHEN THE TESTICLES DO NOT DESCEND INTO THE SCROTUM (CRYPTORCHIDISM)

As a male fetus grows, the testicles begin to form in the fetal abdomen during weeks 6 to 12 of the pregnancy. Before the baby is born, the testicles will slide down the *inguinal canals* (channels in each side of the groin) and into the pouch of skin called the scrotum. A newborn boy's testicles work actively, producing high levels of the hormone testosterone during the first six months of life. This testosterone surge is triggered by the pituitary gland at the base of the brain, which produces a messenger hormone, luteinizing hormone (LH). This hormone tells the testicles to make testosterone (see chapter 4). Testosterone production in the first months of life helps set the stage for normal sperm production later in life.

Testosterone levels tend to be unusually low during infancy in boys with undescended testicles. By the age of 9 months, less than 1 percent of baby boys have one or two undescended testicles (i.e., the testicles remain in the abdomen or groin area instead of in the scrotum). Nowadays, undescended testicles are usually treated when babies are between the ages of 9 and 18 months. Sometimes an extra dose of messenger hormones will stimulate the testicles to descend. More often, surgery is done to bring the baby's testicles down the inguinal canals and into the scrotum. The surgeon frees up the testicle from the surrounding tissues and creates a pocket for it in the scrotum. A stitch may also be added to fix the testicle in the correct position in the scrotum so it cannot retract upward again.

Sometimes, when testicles are high in the abdomen, it is difficult to relocate them into the scrotum. A boy may need two or more operations to complete this task. Rarely, the testicle is removed completely. Some of these testicles are very abnormal and unlikely to produce either hormones or sperm cells if brought into the scrotum. A testis that remains in the abdomen or inguinal canal is a health risk, because it is more likely than a normal testicle to develop testicular cancer as the boy grows to young adulthood and is very difficult to examine. A man's usual lifetime risk of testicular cancer is 1 in 50,000, but if he has had an undescended testicle, his risk increases to about five to nine times that of a man without cryptorchidism. Just as young women are taught breast self-examination to identify abnormal lumps or bumps, every man should start in his teenage years to check his testicles monthly by feeling them to detect changes, such as a lump or a thickening, that could signal a tumor. Pamphlets on how to examine your testicles are available from the American Cancer Society or your doctor's office.

The mature testicle is designed to produce sperm at a temperature slightly below that of the rest of the body. The temperature of a normal testicle is about 93.2° Fahrenheit (plus or minus 3 degrees), compared to a core body temperature averaging 98.6°F (or averages of 34° Celsius for the testicle versus 37°C for the body, for all of you metric fans). When a testicle stays in the abdomen or inguinal canal, the Leydig cells that produce testosterone are not damaged, but the sperm-producing cells can be significantly affected. Some men with undescended testicles will have very poor to no sperm formation as adults, even when they are brought down into the scrotum.

Only in the last 20 years or so have pediatric urologists and surgeons been operating on boys with undescended testicles in infancy. Earlier in the 20th century, boys generally only had surgery later in childhood. Some never had surgery at all because the undescended testicle (usually only on one side in these cases) was never noticed until the boy had his first physical examination for athletics at school.

Since boys who had surgery early in life are just now reaching adulthood, it remains to be seen whether bringing the testicle(s) into the scrotum earlier will improve men's fertility or decrease their risk of testicular cancer—a tumor that occurs most often between the ages of 20 and 40 years.

When only one testicle fails to descend, some recent research suggests that a man's fertility as an adult may be improved if he has surgery before age two to bring it into the scrotum. Other studies, however, have found little influence of age at surgery on a man's ultimate ability to father a child. There is also controversy about how much influence one undescended testicle has in reducing men's fertility. One recent study found that about 10 percent of men with one undescended testicle treated in childhood with surgery had trouble fathering a child, compared to 5 percent of men with normal testicles. Studies clearly agree that infertility is quite common in men who had both testicles undescended. Some of these men have lowered sperm counts and motility. A smaller group have very few or no sperm cells in their semen, but may have small islands of sperm cell production in their testicles, allowing possible surgical sperm retrieval for in vitro fertilization with intracytoplasmic sperm injection (IVF-ICSI) (see chapter 16).

WHEN THE URINARY OPENING IS NOT AT THE TIP OF THE PENIS

One of the most common genital birth defects in male infants is called *hypospadias*. The urinary tube, or urethra, does not develop properly all the way to the tip of the penis, but instead is shortened, opening somewhere on the underside of the penile shaft. In mild cases, the opening is near the area where the head of the penis begins to fan out. Men with this type of hypospadias have no major problem with either ejaculation or urination. Sometimes parents will have this problem corrected in infancy for cosmetic reasons, however. Surgical repair is even more common when the urethra opens along the bottom of the midshaft, or even at the base of the penis. When hypospadias is diagnosed at birth, the baby should not be circumcised, since the surgeon will often use the foreskin to reconstruct a longer urethra. Although these repairs have become very sophisticated and successful, some boys develop *strictures* or a narrowing of their urethra years after surgery from scar tissue. A stricture can limit the amount of semen that a man ejaculates, reducing his chance of fathering a child. Strictures can usually be opened by a surgeon by passing a dilating tube into the urethra, or in severe cases, performing a surgical repair.

If hypospadias is severe and not repaired, a young man may have a fertility problem. If the urethral opening is at the base of the penis, the semen may never even get into his partner's vagina at ejaculation. Even when the opening is at midshaft, the semen is deposited into the lower vagina, where acidic discharge can immobilize sperm cells. Only the very deep part of the vagina offers a nonacidic, more alkaline environment that is friendly to sperm. The occasional man who still has severe hypospadias can ejaculate into a container. The semen he produces can then be used to inseminate his partner.

Some boys born with hypospadias also have a mild to severe curvature of the penis because the urethra is underdeveloped. They may not realize anything is unusual until puberty, when they notice their erection has a distinct hook to it. Most commonly, the curve bends the penis downward, and if significant, it makes intercourse uncomfortable for both partners. This curvature is called *congenital chordee*. It can usually be repaired surgically.

Researchers have noticed that the rates of cryptorchidism, hypospadias, and testicular cancer have all been rising for the last 40 to 50 years in some industrialized countries. The reason for this is a mystery, but one theory is that pollutants in the environment that mimic the chemical estrogen are responsible. During the early weeks of pregnancy, a complex series of hormonal changes occur in the fetus. If the correct levels of hormones are not present, the structures of the male organs may not develop fully.

A less common problem, called *epispadias,* occurs when the urethral opening ends up on the upper side of the penis. Epispadias can occur by itself, or as part of a larger problem in which the urinary bladder ends up on the outer wall of the abdomen instead of inside the pelvis at birth. These problems occur during fetal growth if the male organ system does not finish closing along the midline. Surgery is used to repair these problems as early in life as possible. Even after repair, some men born with epispadias end up with a very short penile shaft, and a few also have some or all of their semen go backward into the bladder at the moment of ejaculation (see chapter 13).

PROBLEMS RESTRICTING
THE FLOW OF SEMEN

Injuries to the urethra can occur in a variety of ways. Remember how many times your bike chain broke, dropping you directly onto the crossbar? Biking injuries to the urethra are not so unusual. The urethra can even be injured occasionally when a medical instrument, such as a catheter, is used to drain the bladder during or after surgery. These injuries can cause scar tissue to form, narrowing the urethra and interfering with expulsion of semen at ejaculation. Most of these strictures can be successfully repaired.

After circumcision, a few infants develop a narrowing of the urinary opening itself, called *meatal stenosis*. A small surgery, called a *meatotomy*, opens the tip of the urethra and corrects this problem. A few boys are born with a congenital problem with the urethra. Usually these problems are diagnosed long before puberty because a boy has trouble urinating, with a slow stream or a urinary stream that splashes upward. Occasionally, however, the main symptom in an adult is that semen just dribbles out at orgasm instead of spurting out, or the amount of semen may be unusually small. Then the problem may only be discovered during an evaluation for infertility.

Occasionally the urethra is very much enlarged, or has pockets, called *diverticula*, along its length. These problems are rare, but can interfere with efficient ejaculation of semen.

PROBLEMS WITH THE FORESKIN

There has been a great deal of controversy about whether to routinely circumcise male babies. Although most babies in the United States are still circumcised, there is little medical rationale for the practice. Men who are not circumcised do occasionally develop foreskin problems, however, that can interfere with sexual function and thus, indirectly, with fertility. Some boys have a tight foreskin that will not pull back smoothly to allow erection to occur comfortably. If the foreskin gets chronically irritated, it may tighten so that only a very small opening is left at the tip and the foreskin can no longer pull back at all. Even if the foreskin is not tight, some men get recurring cracking or bleeding in the foreskin, making intercourse painful. In these situations, circumcision as an adult is usually recommended. Although men worry that they will lose some of the sensitivity of the head of the penis after adult circumcision, scientific evidence does not suggest that circumcised men enjoy sex less.

This chapter discussed problems that occur as the male reproductive equipment is just forming in the fetus. Now we will switch gears to talk about infertility that may result from infections that a man encounters during his lifetime.

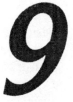

Germs and Germ Cells: Infections and Infertility

In the last chapters we talked about infertility resulting from the bad luck of having something go wrong with your genetic code or your development in the womb. This chapter discusses how germs that you have the misfortune to encounter during your lifetime can interfere with fertility. Some infections that may be linked to infertility include mumps orchitis, tuberculosis, and urethritis. We also describe how the immune system, besides providing the body's infection defenses, can contribute to infertility.

MUMPS ORCHITIS: A BLAST OF THE PAST

Were you a young child before 1967, when the mumps vaccine was introduced? If so, you may remember your mom asking you to go play with your friend Johnny, who had the mumps. Parents wanted their sons to have mumps before the age of puberty. When teens or grown men contract this virus, there is at least a 20 percent chance that not only the parotid glands in their face will swell, but one or both of their testicles may enlarge painfully and grotesquely. You do not need to wonder if you have ever had testicular involvement, or *mumps orchitis*. If you had it, you would remember it! Many men who had mumps orchitis recover and continue to have normal sperm counts and motility. Others may have scarring and shrinkage (atrophy) of the testicle on one or both sides, and permanent problems with sperm quality. In some men, low sperm counts after mumps orchitis are related to blockages in the sperm passageways, and can be improved by microsurgery (see chapter 10). In a minority, however, both testicles are affected and the scarring from the infection is so severe that the seminiferous tubules no longer produce many sperm cells or the motility is very poor. These men are often candidates for in vitro fertilization with intracytoplasmic sperm injection, or IVF-ICSI (see chapter 16). Sometimes their sperm cells may need to be retrieved surgically from the tissue of the testicle itself.

Luckily, this once common childhood disease has become a rarity in the United States. In 1968, 152,209 cases were reported, compared to 1,692 in 1993. We still see cases of men infertile from mumps orchitis coming from less-developed countries, however.

TUBERCULOSIS:
A SCOURGE OF THE PAST REEMERGES

In contrast to mumps, tuberculosis is a disease that has reared its ugly head again in our inner cities, after decades in which we thought we had conquered it. Tuberculosis can cause inflammation of the epididymis, resulting in obstruction of sperm pathways. In more severe cases, it can also destroy some of the sperm-producing tissues of the testis. We only rarely see men infertile because of tuberculosis. Usually they come from third world countries. Unfortunately, some American men afflicted with tuberculosis do not seek treatment for infertility because they are also HIV-positive, or simply cannot afford health care.

HIV-POSITIVE:
CAN A MAN SAFELY FATHER A CHILD?

Men who are infected with the human immunodeficiency virus (HIV) and have partners who are HIV-negative are in a bind. Many of these men will live in relatively good health for a number of years, and the couple may wish to have a child. It may be difficult for them to adopt if the father's HIV status is known. HIV-discordant couples should always practice safer sex, using a condom to prevent exchanging body fluids. Of course, this also prevents pregnancy. Some couples may be comfortable using donor insemination to have a baby, but others want a mutual genetic child. Yet HIV is certainly present in the semen, and there is some evidence that the virus actually sticks to the surface of sperm cells or even lurks inside of them. Even with special sperm-washing techniques (see chapter 16), it would be a risk to the health of mother and potential child to use sperm from an HIV-positive man for intrauterine insemination.

A group in Barcelona, Spain, however, has reported on 63 HIV-positive men who wanted to father a child with their HIV-negative female partners. A very sensitive test for the virus was used on their semen samples, after the sperm cells had been separated out of the seminal fluid and placed in a sterile, nutrient solution instead. Only 6 percent of sperm samples still contained HIV, and these were discarded. The rest of the time, intrauterine insemination was performed with hormone stimulation to promote ovulation for the woman, resulting in 31 pregnancies out of 101 cycles. Thirty-seven babies were born. Nine months later, the women were tested for HIV and none were infected. The babies were also free of infection. Even these techniques are not foolproof, however, and any woman attempting pregnancy in this situation must understand that she is taking a risk of infecting both herself and her unborn child with HIV.

Similar techniques of preparing sperm could potentially be used to select some for IVF-ICSI. This technique would be more expensive, and exposes the woman to more risk of hormones, but minimizes her exposure to HIV.

STDs: JUST SEXUALLY TRANSMITTED DISEASES OR SPERM-TERMINATING DISEASES?

Sexually transmitted diseases (STDs) such as syphilis, gonorrhea, or human immunodeficiency virus have spread around the world, occasionally decimating whole nations in the process. Scientists wonder now if some of the most common STDs of our time—gonorrhea, chlamydia, and ureaplasma urolyticum—may be responsible in part for reports of declining sperm counts in industrialized nations. All three of these bacteria can infect the urethra, causing similar symptoms: pain with urination and ejaculation and a drippy discharge from the urethra. When men have such an infection, called *urethritis,* the culprit is gonorrhea 20 percent of the time. Of the remaining 80 percent of infections, a third to a half are due to an organism called chlamydia, 10 percent to 40 percent to a sub-bacterial organism called ureaplasma, and 20 percent to 30 percent do not show a positive culture at all. Other types of bacteria can also cause urethritis. (Although genital herpes and genital warts are also sexually transmitted, they are caused by a virus, not a bacteria, and do not cause urethritis.)

Tests for chlamydia, mycoplasma, and ureaplasma have improved quite a bit in recent years, now using technology called a *polymerase chain reaction,* or PCR, to detect the genetic code of the bacteria. Once a culture is positive, urethritis can and should be treated with antibiotics, although some strains of gonorrhea have become very stubborn and resistant to all but the strongest drugs. Both the man and his current sexual partner should have cultures and, if positive, be treated with antibiotics. When prescribed an antibiotic, you should always take it as directed, not skipping doses or taking less than the whole amount. If you attack a bacteria with an antibiotic, but then give it a rest by not taking part of the prescription, the bacteria can regroup its defenses, mutating and developing drug resistance. Then a new, more powerful antibiotic will be needed to destroy it. Until an infection is definitely cured, a man and his partner should use condoms to prevent any further contagion to each other.

If a urethral infection remains untreated, it can spread to the epididymis and testicles, causing painful inflammation and damaging the tiny tubules where sperm cells are manufactured and stored. Although the pain of *epididymitis* (an inflammation of the epididymis) often feels like it is limited to one testicle, studies show that the tissue damage from the infection often occurs on both sides. There is yet no proof that STDs cause male infertility, but the evidence is mounting. Sexually transmitted diseases can obstruct the sperm pathways because the inflammation from the infection creates scarring (see the next chapter). One recent study pointed out another connection between STDs and infertility: although men whose antibody testing showed evidence of past infection with chlamydia did not have poorer semen quality, their female partners were more likely to have had pelvic infections that could damage their fallopian tubes.

WHAT DO WHITE CELLS IN THE SEMEN MEAN?

It is not uncommon for men who have absolutely no symptoms of urethritis or other infection to give a semen sample for analysis and get the news that an abnormally high number of white cells have been found in the fluid. Is this evidence of an active infection? All men have some white blood cells in their semen. Test values of less than 1 million white cells for each milliliter of fluid are considered normal. White blood cells are part of the body's immune system, acting as garbage men by eating up foreign bacteria, viruses, or waste products found in the blood or lymph fluid. There is only cause for concern if an excess number of white cells is found in the semen. Furthermore, there is one special type of white cell, called a *granulocyte,* that signals a problem. Granulocytes increase when there is infection or inflammation in an area of the body.

As we discussed in chapter 5, if you have a positive test for white cells, make sure the laboratory is experienced with semen analysis for male infertility. Some laboratories are not very accurate in counting the number of white cells in semen. When testing is done correctly, excess numbers of white cells are found in as many as 1 out of 6 men. What is the source of these white cells? They are almost always from the prostate gland. When white cells are found in the semen, a urologist should also check the fluid secreted from the prostate for white cells. A few drops of this fluid will appear at the opening of the urethra when a physician puts a finger in a man's rectum and gently massages the prostate. This is a mildly uncomfortable and perhaps embarrassing examination, but a helpful one. If the prostate fluid contains excess white cells, the gland itself may be inflamed or infected. For most patients, the first line of defense is to prescribe antibiotics that are effective for prostate infections. Acute prostate infections are fairly rare and very easy to recognize. A man will run a high fever and have intense pain on urination, with ejaculation, or at other times in the area around the prostate. A few men will have chronic bacterial prostatitis that does not have many symptoms.

A large study of 1,710 men in couples being treated for infertility found that as the concentration of white cells in the semen increased, men were more likely to have poor sperm counts and abnormally shaped sperm. This was especially true if over 2 million white cells per milliliter were seen. Some of the men with abnormal numbers of white cells agreed to enter a study in which men would be randomly divided into three groups. The first group would have no treatment and each of the two other groups would be treated with a different antibiotic given to both partners in a couple. Surprisingly, white cell counts decreased by about the same amount in all three groups, suggesting that the antibiotics were not having any real impact. Other studies have found that antibiotics worked for some men, however. One such study in Japan reported the best results when men not only took antibiotics, but also made sure to ejaculate at least once every three days. Frequent ejaculation may somehow reduce inflammation in the prostate.

White cells are often signals not of a prostate infection, but of some inflammation of the prostate tissue. The causes of such inflammation are not well understood. Antibiotics will not get rid of white cells in this case, but having regular ejaculations two or three times a week may help. The hope is that reducing the white cell count will also allow the sperm count and motility to normalize. White cells promote the process of oxidation in nearby sperm cells. Although some oxidation is normal in the body, too much may damage sperm cells, so that they are unable to swim well or to fertilize an egg. Sperm cells and white blood cells produce chemicals that are by-products of oxidation, called *reactive oxygen species* (ROS). When ROS levels are above normal, oxidation is too high. ROS levels can be tested directly.

Decreasing the white cell count in the semen may reduce ROS levels. Another way to counteract ROS may be to use *antioxidant therapy*. Antioxidants include vitamin E (alphatocopherol) and vitamin C (ascorbic acid). Some recent studies suggest that if men have abnormal semen quality, their fertility may improve if they take oral antioxidants. Other scientists are skeptical, however, that these vitamins get into the seminal fluid. More research is needed to see which men may respond to vitamin supplements, and to test whether adding these vitamins by changing one's diet or taking them in the form of a vitamin pill is safer and more effective. For suggestions on getting adequate amounts of vitamins, see chapter 15. Women who may consider trying a dose of antioxidant vitamins along with their mates should be aware that taking more than the daily recommended dose of these vitamins can damage female fertility or cause birth defects if a woman is pregnant.

WHAT IF YOU SEE BLOOD IN YOUR SEMEN?

A few men notice that when they ejaculate their semen has a reddish or brownish tinge, or is frankly bloody. Blood in the semen is called *hematospermia*. Although it often frightens a man to see hematospermia, it rarely is a sign of something serious. It may be due to a broken blood vessel along the semen transport system, or another minor problem, and clears up in a few days. Sometimes it is associated with a prostate infection or, occasionally in older men, with other prostate problems including, though rarely, prostate cancer.

Even though most cases of hematospermia are self-limited, you should notify your doctor when it occurs and then let her or him decide if further investigation is needed. We believe that hematospermia should be evaluated by examining a urine sample for blood or infection, examining the prostate, and testing a semen sample for signs of infection.

If hematospermia persists and no infection has been found, an ultrasound examination of the prostate and seminal vesicles is recommended. In most cases, nothing abnormal is found. The hematospermia may be a sign of temporary inflammation or injury, and, like a nosebleed, will stop on its own. If there is a good deal of blood in your semen, it could affect sperm function. More often, however, a couple's concern is the woman's emotional upset at having bloody semen inside of her vagina after intercourse. Couples may cope with this aesthetic issue by using condoms. Of course, condoms should also be used if a man is at risk for HIV, since the blood in his semen could increase the chances of infecting his partner.

ANTISPERM ANTIBODIES: WHEN THE BODY'S DEFENSES CAUSE INFERTILITY

When George and Janice decided to marry, they agreed to have a child together. George had had a previous vasectomy, so he went ahead and scheduled surgery to reverse it. Within several months, his sperm count was within the usual limits but motility was very low. Most of the sperm clumped together tail to tail. The others just meandered around, without direction. The surgeon told the couple to spend the next six months having intercourse at midcycle, and return only if a pregnancy did not occur. When the happy event never materialized, they did make a new appointment with the infertility specialist. Tests showed that George's sperm were loaded with antibodies. After some soul-searching, the couple decided to try IVF-ICSI, although the reversal surgery had already depleted their bank account. Since Janice was only 29 and had no known infertility problem, she responded very well to the stimulating drugs, producing 16 mature eggs. After ICSI, 10 embryos formed. Two were transferred to Janice's uterus and she became pregnant.

Sometimes a man's body treats his own sperm cells as if they were foreign invaders. His immune system manufactures a defensive system, called antibodies, against his own sperm. These *antisperm antibodies* are like chemicals that stick to the surface of his sperm cells and can hinder their ability to swim or to fertilize an egg.

Antibodies to sperm can form when the barrier between the bloodstream and the sperm-manufacturing portion of the testicle is broken down. Normally, sperm cells from the testis do not get into the bloodstream, where the immune system would react to them. In some cases, such as after a vasectomy, parts of unused sperm cells collect in the testes and can be absorbed into the blood, sometimes sending an alarm to the immune system. Antisperm antibodies form in about half of men after a vasectomy. They may also form if the sperm pathways are obstructed for other reasons (see the next chapter), after infections of or injuries to the epididymis or testicle, or even in men who have a varicocele or a history of an undescended testicle. About 3 percent to 10 percent of men with infertility have antisperm antibodies, some for no clear reason.

Antisperm Antibody Testing. A person's blood, semen, sperm, and even cervical mucus can be tested for antisperm antibodies. Most commonly, the semen and sperm are examined. A variety of tests have been developed and now are standardized and available in most laboratories that perform semen analysis. Some antisperm antibodies cause sperm to clump together (called *agglutination*) so that they get sidetracked along the sperm transport pathways, with fewer and fewer sperm available to reach the egg. In some men, antisperm antibodies interfere with the sperm's ability to swim through the cervical mucus. Antibodies can also prevent sperm from binding to the shell (zona pellucida) of the egg, so that fertilization cannot take place.

It is important to know, however, that having antisperm antibodies in your semen does not always mean you will have a fertility problem. The impact of the antibodies depends on their type, and more importantly, their level or titer; that is, how much of an antibody is present and how active it is.

Treating Infertility Associated with Antisperm Antibodies. Treatments for infertility in men with antisperm antibodies have been varied, and at times controversial. One of the earliest treatments recommended was to use condoms during intercourse. You may well wonder how this was supposed to aid in conceiving a child! We may laugh now, but at the time the theory was that lessening the woman's exposure to her partner's sperm would decrease the amounts of antisperm antibodies in her system, making her cervical mucus more receptive. After six months of using a condom, the couple was instructed to "go for it," and have unprotected intercourse at midcycle. Unfortunately, theory did not translate well into success. For one thing, this method did nothing to decrease antisperm antibodies in the man's own semen.

Among other techniques tried, one of the most debated was using *corticosteroids* (cortisone) to suppress the immune response which causes antibodies to form. Some physicians used high doses of steroids briefly, whereas others preferred low doses prescribed for longer periods. Although these medications were used widely, overall the research showed that men did not respond consistently to them. Unfortunately, corticosteroids can also have a number of unpleasant and even dangerous side effects (acne, facial swelling, reduced resistance to infection, and occasionally damage to joints) that may override their potential usefulness in fertility treatment.

Currently, the most common way of treating men with antisperm antibodies is to use assisted reproductive techniques (ART), as we describe in chapter 16. One approach has been to try to "wash off" the antibodies with special sperm preparation techniques, but this is far easier said than done. The antibody attaches firmly to the sperm cell. Even multiple washings of sperm may not decrease antibody levels. At best, any sperm free of antibodies will be isolated and can be used for insemination.

If a pregnancy does not result from insemination, IVF may be considered. As we mentioned before, some antibodies can actually interfere with fertilization. In this case, conventional IVF might not work either. In vitro fertilization with ICSI can bypass this problem, since the sperm does not have to bind to the zona pellucida. Instead, the sperm is injected directly into the interior of the egg. IVF-ICSI appears to work very well in overcoming infertility related to antisperm antibodies.

If a couple is trying to decide with their doctors whether to use conventional IVF versus IVF-ICSI, tests revealing antisperm antibodies may tilt the scale toward the ICSI side, in order to avoid the wasted time and money of a failed IVF cycle. It is important to remember, however, that not all antibodies interfere with the fertilization step. Some of the more sophisticated tests of sperm function described in chapter 5 may also be helpful in deciding on the most effective treatment option. Other factors that enter into the decision could include the degree of sperm agglutination, the number of motile sperm, whether fertilization had failed in a previous IVF cycle, and the cost difference (about $1,000 in most centers) to perform ICSI.

10

The Boulder on the Path: Obstructive Infertility

In Stuttgart, Germany, workers use state-of-the-art equipment to build the Mercedes automobile, arguably one of the finest production cars in the world. Once made, these expensive vehicles are sent by train, boat, and truck to be taken to their final destination and used. Without a proper transportation system, however, they would sit in the factory, eventually rusting and disintegrating from disuse. Similarly, a blockage anywhere along the human sperm transport system (including the rete testes, efferent ducts, epididymis, vas deferens, and ejaculatory ducts) will prevent perfectly good sperm from leaving the body. Like the Mercedes, these stored sperm will ultimately age, disintegrate, and disappear.

ROADBLOCKS TO SPERM TRANSPORT

Sperm can be blocked from traveling their natural pathway for many reasons. The typical cause is scar tissue from an infection or injury. The most common kind of infection causing obstruction is a painful inflammation of the epididymis, called epididymitis. When a vasectomy is performed, the vas deferens is cut on purpose, creating a permanent blockage.

The vas deferens may also be trapped or inadvertently cut during an operation such as a hernia repair, a kidney transplant, or other surgery performed in the groin area or deep in the pelvis where the vas deferens heads towards the prostate gland. The most common surgical injury occurs when an infant has surgery to repair an inguinal hernia, an abnormal bulge of muscle in the groin area. The vas deferens is extremely small and delicate at that age. Even when the surgeon takes the greatest care, an injury can occur. Luckily, most infants, children, or young adults who have hernia repairs have no injury to their reproductive equipment. If you are having an infertility workup, however, and know you had a hernia repair, be sure to mention it to your doctor.

When both testicles are blocked, there are usually clear signs. No sperm will be found in the seminal fluid which is ejaculated at orgasm. If only one side is scarred or cut and the opposite side is open, a man may never know that anything is amiss unless sperm production becomes poor in the unobstructed testicle. Then, infertility may result.

SHOOTING BLANKS:
SEMEN WITHOUT SPERM CELLS

You may wonder why semen still flows out at ejaculation if sperm transport is blocked. In most cases, the blockage only affects the route of the sperm cells from the testicles where they are manufactured. The fluid making up semen is made in the prostate and seminal vesicles (see chapter 4 for more detail). These glands usually remain unblocked.

The amount of fluid that comes out at orgasm will only be notably reduced if there is a blockage where the tubes of the ejaculatory ducts come through the prostate (see Fig. 10.1). Even in this situation, a small amount of fluid, produced within the prostate itself, is still available at the moment of orgasm. If the vas deferens (the tube bringing sperm cells from the testicle) is blocked before it joins the seminal vesicles, the volume of semen is not noticeably less, since only about 5 percent of semen comes from the testicles, epididymis, and vas deferens.

HOW DOES YOUR DOCTOR
FIND AN OBSTRUCTION?

For the most part, finding an obstruction in the epididymis, vas deferens, or ejaculatory ducts is fairly routine. If the doctor suspects a blockage, there are specific tests that will heighten the suspicion and others

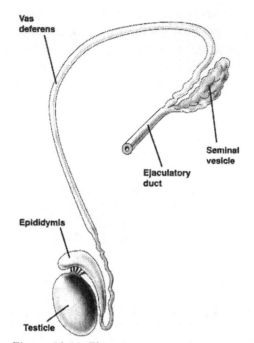

Figure 10.1   The sperm transport system

that ultimately can prove it. Often, the location of the blockage can be pinpointed, allowing the possibility of surgery to fix it.

Usually the blockage causes the "red flag" of infertility, which leads you to seek medical help to begin with. More rarely, a man feels actual discomfort in his testicles. When the doctor examines you, he may notice thickening of the epididymis and or vas deferens, which becomes swollen and filled with trapped sperm or decayed sperm parts. These areas may also feel tender when they are pressed. Yet the testicles are normal in size and texture. A semen analysis would reveal that there are no sperm cells.

It is particularly important for the doctor to accurately identify all the elements of the sperm transport system, since one or more parts could be absent from birth. For example, as we discussed in chapter 7, in two out of every hundred men who have no sperm in their semen, the vas deferens never developed, so there was no way for sperm to naturally exit the testicle. Careful examination can *usually* identify whether a vas deferens is present on one or both sides.

After the physical examination, the doctor may ask for another semen analysis, depending on the number and the type of semen tests done beforehand. Not only are the number of sperm cells in the semen important, but it is also necessary to check for sperm cells in a sample of urine that a man produces immediately after ejaculating. Some men do not have an obstruction of sperm transportation, but instead ejaculate all or almost all of their semen backward into the bladder, rather than outward through the penis at the moment of climax. This condition is called *retrograde ejaculation* and is discussed fully in chapter 13.

If all the semen flows out normally, it is a good idea to take a sample and have the laboratory concentrate it by spinning it for a few minutes in a machine called a *centrifuge*. This forces all the cells present in the seminal fluid to form a small pellet in the bottom of a test tube. This material is spread out on a glass microscope slide, stained with special chemicals that help identify certain types of cells, and examined for the presence of sperm. Sometimes sperm will be found in the concentrated pellet, even when it appeared at first that none were in the semen.

Hormone tests are also important to rule out hormonal problems that could cause a lack of sperm cells. The hormone tests typically used to diagnose male infertility are discussed in chapter 5, and hormonal problems that lead to infertility are described in chapter 11.

SURGERY TO REPAIR OBSTRUCTIONS

Once an obstruction is identified, it can often be repaired with surgery. Since a vasectomy creates a man-made obstruction, vasectomy reversal is one of these operations. Other operations use similar techniques to bypass the blocked area. Surgery to correct an obstruction to sperm transport is only worthwhile if enough sperm cells are being made in the testicles. When a semen sample contains very few or no sperm cells, a testicular biopsy is often an important way to examine sperm production directly to help guide treatment planning (see chapter 5).

THROUGH THE LOOKING GLASS: THE INCREDIBLE WORLD OF MICROSURGERY

The procedures used to repair obstructions require the techniques of *microsurgery*, in which the surgeon operates using a special, large microscope to magnify the tiny structures that he or she is repairing. Eye surgeons were the first specialists to recognize the value of micro-

surgery. In the early 1970s, some urologists and plastic surgeons realized that they could accurately reconnect tiny structures in the male
reproductive tract, such as nerves, blood vessels, or tubes in the epididymis, if they used a high degree of magnification to see better. Over
the years large, freestanding operating microscopes were developed,
along with smaller instruments and finer thread used for sewing. This
new technology vastly improved the success of operations to correct
obstructions of sperm transport or to reverse vasectomies.

HOW TO FIND THE BEST
SURGEON FOR MALE INFERTILITY

Just as urologists do not always have specialized training in infertility,
most are not expert in performing microsurgery to repair obstructions
and reverse vasectomies. It takes practice to become really skilled in this
area. A surgeon also will maintain those skills if she or he has the chance
to do the procedures many times a year.

How can you find a urologist expert in microsurgery?

- If you already have a urologist who has diagnosed your infertility, you
  have a right to know about the urologist's training. Did he or she
  have an infertility fellowship, or at least a number of months of specialized training during residency years? How much training and
  experience in microsurgery has your urologist had? If you are planning to have surgery, ask how many microsurgery procedures a year
  your urologist performs. You also have a right to know the pregnancy rates after these surgeries, if that information is available.

- If you do not have a urologist, you need a good referral. You may
  want to ask the gynecologist or reproductive endocrinologist who
  has been helping with an infertility workup, or consult your family
  doctor. You can also call your local county or city's urology association, or call the American Urological Association and ask for urologists in your area who specialize in infertility surgery. If there is a
  medical school near where you live, try calling their Department of
  Urology and finding out if a member of the faculty is trained in
  microsurgery.

- If your insurance coverage includes infertility surgery, but restricts
  you to only certain urologists or medical centers, you may be tempted just to follow the path of least resistance and use the physician

available. Remember that the quality of this surgery will determine your chance to ever achieve a pregnancy. And an operation also carries physical risk and discomfort. You may decide you would be better off paying some or all of the costs out of your own pocket if necessary to have the procedure done by an expert.

MICROSURGERY TO REPAIR A VASECTOMY OR CORRECT A BLOCKAGE

Whether a surgeon is reversing a vasectomy or repairing a blockage in the vas deferens occurring from other causes, similar techniques of microsurgery are used. The operation is called a *vasovasostomy*. It is usually performed in an outpatient setting, so that men can return home the same day, often within hours after the surgery. Several different types of anesthesia can be used, and patient and surgeon should discuss the options ahead of time to choose the safest and most effective one for their particular circumstances. With general anesthesia, the patient is completely unconscious. A regional anesthetic leaves the patient awake, but uses anesthesia placed around the spinal column, numbing the patient from the waist down. A local anesthetic is a third option, injecting an anesthetic drug with a fine needle directly into the area of the surgery to numb the tissue. Often, sedative drugs are given along with the local anesthesia to make the patient comfortable and fully relaxed.

Vasovasostomy involves making an incision in the scrotum just large enough to allow the surgeon to find the vas deferens and identify the blocked area or the site of a previous vasectomy. The vas deferens is a muscular tube with a diameter of about 1/8 inch. In its middle, a tiny channel forms the sperm cells' highway. The surgeon will remove the scar tissue from both ends of the vas deferens. Two freshly cut ends of the tube are left. The two small openings must be precisely aligned and carefully sewn together without any leaks, and with a technique that should prevent excessive scar tissue from forming during healing. Once sewn together, the vas deferens is placed back into the scrotum and the incision is sewn closed.

Sometimes after vasectomy the vas deferens is not the *only* sperm pathway that is obstructed, and reconnecting its two ends will not remove all the roadblocks in the sperm transport system. Another area of blockage that can occur is in the delicate epididymis, the coiled tube

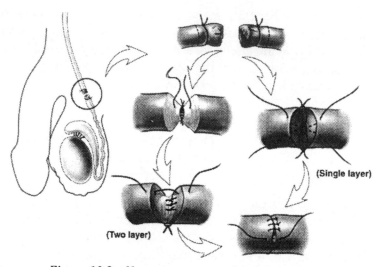

Figure 10.2   Vascectomy reversal (vasovasostomy)

that lies against the testicle where sperm cells mature. This happens more commonly when the vasectomy had been performed many years previously. Over the years, more sperm may be produced than the body can absorb, increasing the pressure inside the epididymis and vas deferens. The result is a blowout much like the leak that occurs in the weakest spot of an overinflated tire. This blowout can only be identified at the time of surgery.

The epididymis may also develop a blockage as a result of infection or injury. Occasionally, a man is born with a blockage. Whatever the reason, the surgical procedure to bypass the epididymal blockage remains the same. The epididymis is carefully examined and samples of fluid are taken, first from its most distant end (furthest from the testicle and closest to the vas deferens). If no sperm are found, the tube is sampled again, closer and closer to its top, until sperm are found. This is the site where the end of the vas deferens will be connected to the epididymis.

To bypass the blockage in the epididymis, the surgeon must connect the upper portion of the vas deferens to the correct area of the epididymis itself (see Fig. 10.3). This type of surgery is even more technically demanding, because the tubules that make up the epididymis are even smaller and thinner than the vas deferens. The success rate for this type of surgery, called a *vasoepididymostomy,* depends on several factors, including the experience of the surgeon and the location of the blockage. The closer to the top (or testicle) that the new connection is

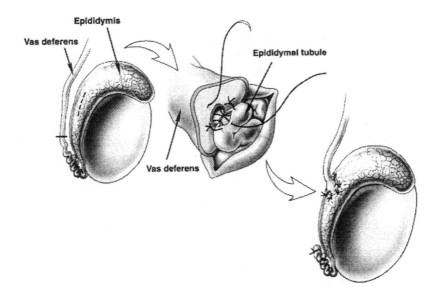

Figure 10.3   Creating a vasoepididymostomy

made, the less mature the sperm will be. Consequently the pregnancy rate will be lower.

HOW SUCCESSFUL IS VASECTOMY REVERSAL?

Many men would like information about the success of reversing a vasectomy. Millions of men have had voluntary vasectomies, thinking their family was complete or that they never wished to have children. Circumstances change, however, and sometimes men regret the decision they made in the past. The most common scenario is when a man remarries and would like to have children with his new wife.

Men often underestimate the success rates of vasectomy reversal. The chances of getting sperm cells flowing again, and more important-ly, achieving a pregnancy, depend on a number of elements. The skill of the surgeon is paramount, but aside from that, one of the most impor-tant factors is the length of time that has passed since the original vasec-tomy. In a study published in 1991 that included some of our own patients and those of four other urologists with equal skill in micro-surgery, the success rates were extremely high when the reversal was done within 3 years after the vasectomy: 97 percent of men had sperm in their semen again and 76 percent were able to get their wives pregnant. If it had been 3 to 8 years since the vasectomy, 88 percent of men had sperm in the semen and 53 percent established a pregnancy. If the vasectomy had been done between 9 and 14 years before, 45 percent fathered a pregnancy. When the vasectomy was more than 14 years old, however, the pregnancy rate dropped to 30 percent. All but the lowest of these rates are higher, however, than the typical success of a cycle of in vitro fertilization using sperm injection. Another advantage is that vasectomy reversal spares a woman with normal fertility from undergoing the medical risks of IVF.

NONSURGICAL OPTIONS FOR OBSTRUCTION

The success of IVF-ICSI has opened up a new range of options for men with obstruction of the sperm pathways. Sperm can be retrieved directly from the epididymis or even from the tissue of the testicle itself. Although these sperm cells are not numerous enough, or do not have good enough motility to use for intrauterine insemination or conventional IVF, they are sufficient for IVF-ICSI. In chapter 23, we compare the cost-effectiveness of some of these treatment options for obstruction.

11

Is It My Hormones?

Whenever we think of infertility, we think about hormones. Although they are just the chemical messengers that tell the reproductive organs what to do, hormones seem mysterious and complex. If they are out of balance, perhaps they are interfering with fertility. This speculation also carries the hope that restoring hormonal balance could improve a man's chances of fathering a child. In fact, hormonal causes of male infertility are relatively uncommon. When they do occur, however, some can be effectively treated. Therefore it is important to understand them and have hormone tests done when it is appropriate.

Let's quickly review again how hormones control sperm production in men. You may want to glance back at the diagram of the hormone system on page 30. Remember that the hypothalamus produces the messenger hormone gonadotropin-releasing hormone (GnRH), which tells the pituitary gland to make the right amounts of follicle-stimulating hormone (FSH) and luteinizing hormone (LH). Follicle-stimulating hormone acts directly on the cells of the testicles responsible for sperm production, and LH controls the testosterone-producing cells. This system usually works quite well, but as you can imagine, it can occasionally get out of whack in a variety of ways.

WHEN THE CAPTAIN IS ASLEEP AT THE HELM

Some men are born with or develop a problem in which the hypothalamus fails to produce GnRH. Called *hypothalamic-hypogonadotropic-*

hypogonadism, this problem is similar to having a ship without a competent captain. The signal is never sent to the pituitary, and so LH and FSH are not produced. The testicles remain turned off and fail to produce testosterone or sperm cells. This type of problem is rare, but can be the result of a developmental error.

Some of the structures in the hypothalamus never develop correctly in the fetus. Men with this problem (referred to as *Kallman's syndrome,* named after Dr. Franz Kallman, who first described it) also sometimes lack a sense of smell or may be born with other problems such as cleft palate, undescended testicles, or deafness. Sometimes Kallman's syndrome is inherited, but not always. It is often not diagnosed until a boy fails to go through the physical changes of puberty. Men with Kallman's syndrome can be treated with hormones that replace the GnRH, and may then regain normal fertility. Some other, even rarer genetic conditions also involve failure of the hypothalamus to develop.

WHEN THE FIRST MATE
DOES NOT FOLLOW ORDERS

You can think of the pituitary gland as the first mate on the hormone ship. The pituitary is supposed to take commands from the captain (the hypothalamus), and relay them to the testicular crew. The pituitary can be damaged by an injury, as a side effect of brain surgery or radiation to treat a brain tumor, or if a tumor grows in the pituitary gland itself. Once in a great while the pituitary simply fails to produce LH or FSH. When this occurs, the missing hormones can be replaced to restore fertility.

The most common primary pituitary problem involved in male infertility, however, is termed *hyperprolactinemia,* an overproduction of the hormone *prolactin.* In women, prolactin stimulates milk production in the breasts. In men, it plays a role in sperm production. Men occasionally develop tumors in the pituitary that produce large amounts of prolactin—often several hundred times the normal level found in the bloodstream. The great majority of these tumors are benign (i.e., not cancerous), and do not spread to other areas of the body. If a tumor is allowed to grow unchecked, however, it can eventually damage the structures close to it, such as the optic nerve. A growing pituitary tumor can cause headaches, significant visual problems, and even blindness.

Symptoms of a prolactin-secreting tumor include diminished sperm counts, loss of sexual desire, trouble reaching orgasm, growing breast tissue around the nipples, and occasionally having clear fluid drip from the nipples.

Prolactin-secreting pituitary tumors can be diagnosed with special imaging techniques, such as *magnetic resonance imaging* (MRI) or *computerized tomographic X rays* (CT scans). Occasionally radiation or surgery is used to treat a very large tumor, but most shrink with medication. Bromocriptine (Parlodel) is the most common medication used for this condition, though nausea is a fairly frequent side effect. Other medications (for example, cabergolamine or quinagolide) can also be used if bromocriptine is not successful or is poorly tolerated. When the prolactin level decreases, other hormones and sperm production often improve.

WHEN THE CREW
CAN'T RESPOND TO ORDERS

Sometimes the hypothalamus and the pituitary give all the right commands, but regardless of the amount of pituitary hormones produced, the testicles fail to respond with more testosterone and/or sperm cells. Some of these problems are caused by genetic abnormalities, quirks of fate in a man's normal pattern of 46, XY chromosomes. For example, as we discuss in chapter 7, men with the genetic variation of Klinefelter syndrome have not just an X and a Y chromosome, but two Xs and a Y. Men with Klinefelter's have small testicles, but usually produce enough testosterone to have normal sexual desire and function. In some men with genetic abnormalities, a little sperm production may occur somewhere within the small testicles. Sometimes a few sperm cells can be retrieved from the tissue of these testicles and used for IVF-ICSI (in vitro fertilization with intracytoplasmic sperm injection). A son born from these procedures would have a possibility of inheriting the same genetic problem that his father has, however.

There are other reasons unrelated to genetics for the testicles being unable to respond to the pituitary gland's orders. If the testicles sustained a severe infection, such as mumps orchitis (see chapter 9), or were exposed to radiation or chemotherapy for cancer treatment (see chapter 14), the sperm-producing seminiferous tubules can scar. Sometimes the parent spermatogonia that produce new, immature sperm are simply destroyed. Some men are born with one or both testicles either in the abdomen or groin area. When the testicles do not descend into the scrotum before or shortly after birth, sperm production can also be permanently damaged (see chapter 8).

It is still fairly common to see no sperm cell production, and yet infertility experts remain at a loss to explain why the testicles are failing. As we discussed in chapter 7, recent genetic research has pinpointed some areas on the Y chromosome that are essential for sperm cell production. We can identify the 9 percent to 18 percent of men with very few or no sperm who have missing genetic material in these areas, but that still leaves us in a quandary to explain to other men why their sperm production has halted. Perhaps in the future we will be able to identify other genetic problems that affect spermatogenesis.

WHEN FSH IS HIGH, BUT SPERM PRODUCTION IS LOW

It is not unusual for a man to have very low sperm counts or no sperm in his semen at all, combined with a very high FSH level. The FSH level is a sign of damage in the testicle to the sperm-producing cells. One of the more common diagnoses made in men who have a high level of the hormone FSH and no sperm in their semen is *Sertoli cell only syndrome*. As you may remember from chapter 4, Sertoli cells are a type of "nurse" cell inside the sperm-producing tubules. They nurture the developing sperm cells until they are fully formed and ready to be released to travel to the epididymis and beyond. As the name of the syndrome implies, the tubules contain only Sertoli cells and no parent spermatogonia cells or developing sperm. The Leydig cells, outside of the tubules, produce normal amounts of testosterone, keeping LH levels normal. Without sperm formation, however, there is no feedback mechanism to tell the pituitary to decrease the amount of FSH it produces. The FSH level is usually significantly elevated, as the pituitary keeps striving to push the testicles to the impossible task of making sperm without the needed raw materials. Thus, the high hormone levels are a healthy response of the man's body to an abnormal situation.

Some men in this category may still have small islands of sperm cell production in their testicular tissue. If these sperm cells can be found and retrieved by taking several testicular biopsies, they can be used for

IVF-ICSI (see chapter 16). The only way to know if any sperm cells exist in the testicles is to actually get a sample of tissue and look for them. The FSH level is not a reliable indicator.

TREATING LOW TESTOSTERONE

Low testosterone can be diagnosed by a routine blood test, although abnormal results are uncommon in healthy men under age 50. It is relatively easy to replace testosterone when the testicles fail to manufacture enough. It can be given effectively in a monthly injection or by wearing a skin patch on the scrotum or the abdomen. Testosterone replacement can restore sexual desire and erections, and may improve fertility if low testosterone was the only obstacle. If your testosterone level is low, your doctor should try to find out the reason, so the problem can be treated in the most effective way. Sometimes replacing testosterone is not the answer, since the low level is a sign of another hormone problem. Correcting that abnormality will automatically also improve testosterone. When the sperm-producing areas of the testicle fail to work, testosterone treatments cannot restore sperm production.

OTHER IMPORTANT
MEMBERS OF THE CREW

Continuing our metaphor, a couple of other hormones are necessary for the ship of fertility to sail. The hormones produced by the thyroid gland can interfere with sperm production if their levels are too high (hyperthyroidism) or too low (hypothyroidism). A few men have a disorder called *acromegaly,* in which the pituitary produces too much human growth hormone. Some of these men also have too much prolactin or too little LH, and their fertility may be affected. Another hormonal syndrome that can affect fertility is *Cushing's syndrome,* in which the adrenal glands produce too much of the stress hormone cortisol. Men with Cushing's syndrome often have lowered LH or testosterone. When these conditions create hormone imbalances, the problem with fertility can often be corrected by using either hormone replacement, medications, or surgery to restore normal hormone levels.

HORMONES AND YOUR WEIGHT

Men who are extremely overweight sometimes have poor sperm quality that may be related to their hormone levels. Fatty tissue converts testosterone to estrogenlike chemicals, so that very obese men (for example, men who weigh well over 300 pounds composed mostly of fat) may have normal FSH levels, but an abnormally high ratio of estrogen compared to testosterone. On the other end of the spectrum, some men become anorexic through compulsive diet and exercise. If they become skeletally thin and do not have normal muscle mass, their fertility will also decline, just as it would if a man were starving to death.

PRESCRIPTION MEDICINES THAT CAN AFFECT HORMONES

Some medications you may take for a health problem unrelated to your infertility can unbalance your reproductive hormones. Men with ulcers may take high doses of cimetidine (Tagamet), which can interfere with testosterone levels. Men who have psychiatric disorders such as schizophrenia sometimes take major tranquilizers called phenothiazines, which also can have hormonal side effects. Medicines used to treat depression can also interfere with ejaculation. Men who have had organ transplants may be on an immune-system-suppressing drug, such as cyclosporine or immuran. Your infertility specialist should know about any prescription drugs you may be taking.

IS CLOMIPHENE EVER USEFUL?

Many men with poor semen quality have been dosed with clomiphene citrate (Clomid or Serophene). This is an option to try if a man's hormones are basically all normal, but his sperm count is low, and no obstruction exists to explain the problem. A subgroup of men, perhaps 1 out of 10 in this situation, may have better sperm production if FSH is artificially elevated by using the drug clomiphene citrate. Although there is little strict scientific proof for its usefulness, we have used it on occasion. We closely monitor hormone levels and semen changes while a man is on the drug. If the hormone increases are modest, remaining in the high normal range, we continue the drug for six to nine more months, reevaluating the man's hormones and semen analysis during that time. If there are no positive changes in sperm quality by six months, we stop the drug and go on to other treatments.

OTHER HORMONAL THERAPIES

Other hormonally related treatments are sometimes used to try to rev up sperm cell production. One is the drug tamoxifen (Nolvadex), which is mainly used in the United States to prevent or treat breast cancer. In Europe, however, it is used to treat both female and male infertility. Another is human chorionic gonadotropin (HCG), a pituitary hormone that triggers ovulation in women and is thought to stimulate sperm cell production under some conditions in men. There is even less scientific evidence of the effectiveness of these hormones, except in the rare instance that we can prove that we are replacing depleted natural hormone levels.

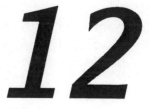

Varioceles: How Important Are They?

A *varicocele* is a cluster of large, dilated veins that drain blood away from one or both of the testicles. All men have veins in this area. A varicocele develops during puberty if the veins lack the small leaflets or valves that keep blood from flowing backward. Varicose veins in the legs usually occur when the valves lose their strength, but with a varicocele, the valves were missing from the outset. The blood still flows toward the heart as it would normally, but when a man stands, the vein fills and blood flow may be a bit sluggish, allowing the vein to stretch.

Most men do not even know they have a varicocele (or sometimes one on each side of the scrotum). Sometimes a physician will point it out during a physical examination. Other times, it is only discovered after an abnormal semen analysis alerts the physician to look for a varicocele. To find the varicocele, the doctor must examine the man's testicles while he is standing upright. When a man lies down flat on his back, the veins tend to collapse. Although you might expect a varicocele to look like the swollen blue canals you would see in a varicose vein on someone's leg, the skin of the scrotum is often thick enough to hide the varicocele. A man would be unlikely to see it, even if he looked carefully in the mirror.

WHY DO VARICOCELES FORM?

You might guess that a varicocele would form if a man did heavy manual labor or perhaps lifted weights. You would be wrong, however. About 15 percent of American men develop varicoceles by adulthood. No one understands why they occur in some men and not others. Historically, the first recorded description of a varicocele was by Celsius, a Greek physician in the first century B.C. He not only described the varicocele accurately, but was skilled enough to notice that in some men the affected testicle (usually the left) was smaller than its opposite partner.

HOW DO VARICOCELES
AFFECT FERTILITY?

Despite the fact that varicoceles have been recognized for 2,000 years, we still do not completely understand why they interfere with sperm quality. Indeed, some men with varicoceles have excellent semen quality and establish pregnancies without a problem. Others can have anything from mild to severe problems with their fertility. There are several current theories regarding why a varicocele impacts on fertility.

It is no accident that the testicles hang in the scrotal pouch below a man's abdomen. They function best in a cooler environment. If the testicles are exposed to the normal body temperature of 98.6°F, sperm formation stops. In the scrotum, the temperature is about 4 or 5 degrees cooler. Research suggests that a varicocele increases the temperature of the testicle, not necessarily to the point of stopping sperm production, but enough at times to change the process. As a result, fewer sperm cells are manufactured, and those that do mature may be less motile (i.e., less powerful swimmers) or misshapen.

Another theory is that a varicocele may cause a harmful backflow of chemicals from the adrenal gland on the same side. The adrenal glands sit on top of each kidney and produce hormones that help the body cope with physical and emotional stress. The veins draining blood concentrated with stress hormones from the adrenal glands lie just above the veins draining the testicle. A varicocele may allow the testicles to get a hefty dose of these chemicals. Other researchers have focused on the idea that blood pooling in the enlarged veins no longer delivers a healthy amount of oxygen to the sperm-producing areas of the testicle. More recent experiments, however, show that a varicocele actually results in an increase in the blood flow to a testicle. The result, though, is an increase in temperature, probably accounting for the decrease in sperm quality.

Obviously, our knowledge about varicoceles is far from complete. Some experts still believe that varicoceles are not a major cause of infertility. Despite the ongoing controversy, we think the evidence does point to varicoceles as a cause of infertility in some men. In 1992, the World Health Organization sponsored a study to determine the impact of varicoceles on semen quality. Members of an international study group examined over 9,000 men in couples with infertility. Twenty-five percent of men with abnormal semen analyses had a varicocele, compared to only 11 percent of those who had normal sperm quality.

WHEN SHOULD
A VARICOCELE BE TREATED?

About 15 percent of men have a varicocele. Many of these men have no known problems with fertility. In recent years, specialists have disagreed, sometimes passionately, about when or whether a varicocele should be treated. While not every varicocele needs to be corrected, there are situations where getting rid of a varicocele can significantly improve fertility.

Again, a number of studies indicate that destroying varicoceles can improve sperm quality for some men, but others have not found treatment to be effective. Still, there are more studies that weigh in on the positive side. One that we find very compelling was done in Israel. A group of infertile couples in which the husbands had varicoceles was followed for three years. Half of the men had their varicoceles corrected and half were just observed for the first year. Of the men who had varicocele surgery, 44 percent established a pregnancy during the next year, compared to only 10 percent of the men who remained under observation. At the end of the year, the remaining men who had not had surgery were offered the operation. Ultimately, slightly more than two-thirds of men who had surgery got their wives pregnant.

The relationship between having a varicocele and having reduced semen quality is strong, but it is not 100 percent. Each couple must be evaluated for their unique infertility factors. Just because a man has a varicocele does not mean he will have trouble fathering a child. Even if a man has a varicocele and also abnormal semen quality, the varicocele may not always account for the fertility problem. Suspicion should be high that the varicocele is part of the problem, however. Overall, research suggests that about two-thirds of men who have procedures to fix a varicocele improve at least one aspect of their semen quality. About 40 percent ultimately establish a pregnancy.

> Winston and Tiwanna had been married for four years. They waited two years to try for a pregnancy. Only a month after Tiwanna stopped using birth control pills, she became pregnant, but sadly she miscarried six weeks later. The couple took a brief rest and then began trying again to conceive, but after 18 months, a second pregnancy had still not occurred. Frustrated and worried, they consulted an infertility specialist. Tiwanna's examination was normal. She had regular menstrual cycles and appeared to be ovulating. Her uterus and fallopian tubes were healthy. Winston was also found to be in excellent health, but examination of his testicles revealed a moderately large varicocele on the left. Although his left testicle was slightly smaller than the right, its size was still in the normal range. A semen analysis showed a low count (12 million sperm per milliliter of semen) and reduced motility (32 percent). The number of normally shaped sperm (morphology) was also slightly low at 22 percent (30 percent or more is considered normal). Two more semen samples were analyzed, with very similar results. Winston was advised to have his varicocele corrected. Within 6 months, Winston's semen analysis improved markedly. The count rose to 52 million sperm per milliliter of semen with 60 percent motility. In month 7, Tiwanna conceived and ultimately delivered a healthy baby girl.

When a man with a varicocele has excellent sperm quality, it is important to check all possible factors on the female side. Some sophisticated tests of sperm function can also help in treatment planning (see chapter 5). These tests measure how sperm may travel or penetrate an egg after they have been ejaculated. In some men with varicoceles, these tests may uncover unsuspected sperm problems. If the tests continue to be normal, however, correction of a varicocele may not be indicated.

> Steve and Beth were in their mid-30s and had tried for a number of years to get pregnant. Each had undergone infertility testing, including a laparoscopy for Beth, with no abnormal findings. Beth had tried oral medicines to increase ovulation, but still had no

pregnancy. Steve had two semen analyses, but all the numbers checked out in the normal range. He went to a urologist and was found to have a small varicocele. The urologist recommended surgery, but Steve felt hesitant and got a second opinion. This urologist used more sophisticated tests to see how Steve's sperm cells performed under conditions that might mimic conception. Steve's sperm performed like pros in all the tests. Instead of suggesting varicocele surgery, this infertility specialist recommended the couple try intrauterine insemination with Steve's sperm, bypassing some parts of the reproductive cycle that could possibly be problematic. Three cycles later, Beth conceived.

HOW ARE VARICOCELES TREATED?

Most of us are familiar with the kind of varicose veins you would see in someone's legs. They often cause discomfort and sometimes need to be treated. In the past, large varicose veins were treated by surgical removal, called stripping. Today many patients only require nonsurgical treatment—for example, injecting a solution into the veins that will cause them to scar shut. The blood that traveled through those veins is rerouted to deeper, healthier ones. With varicoceles, there was never a thought of stripping the veins out (ouch!!!), but surgeons have learned how to tie the veins off or plug them up from inside.

Just as there are many ways to skin the proverbial cat, there are several methods to get rid of a varicocele. Most procedures are done on an outpatient basis, and are relatively simple and minimally invasive. (Notice that we did not call them minor surgeries, since no surgery that involves a man's genitals should ever be considered minor!) The whole idea is not to remove or strip the veins, but rather to block the blood flow through the veins, forcing it to pass through other, more normal veins that have valves. This avoids the heating effect from having the blood flow through the dilated, abnormal veins.

The most common way of correcting a varicocele is still to use surgery to tie off the dilated veins. The veins are easiest to spot in the scrotum, but the incision is made in the groin area or upper scrotum where many veins join to become few. Those remaining veins are tied off with delicate sutures. In recent years, urologists who are experienced microsurgeons have used the operating microscope to magnify even the smallest veins. This may allow them to effectively tie off all the dilated veins through a smaller incision. Other surgeons still prefer the more standard approach, using a somewhat larger incision in the groin area, similar to one that would be made to repair a hernia.

Women who have gone through infertility testing are often familiar with *laparoscopy,* sometimes called "belly-button surgery," because a thin telescope is inserted into the body through a small opening just below the navel. This type of approach can also be used on men, to tie off the varicocele at the point where the veins enter the muscular opening in the wall of the abdomen. After the patient is given general anesthesia, a thin telescope attached to a camera is inserted through the small incision, followed by two smaller probes that are passed through tiny openings made on each side between the navel and the pubic bone. These probes form a passageway through which surgical instruments can be passed. The surgeon uses these instruments to separate the veins of the varicocele from the artery and lymph vessels. Then the surgeon passes a special stapling tool through one of the small openings and blocks off the veins using stainless steel clips.

There is even a way of correcting a varicocele without making a surgical incision at all. This method is called *transvenous* (i.e., through the vein) *embolization* (i.e., creation of a clot in a vein). Embolization is done by an interventional radiologist who has had special training. The radiologist uses an X-ray viewing screen (fluoroscope) to see the blood vessels in the crucial area. A very thin tube, called a catheter, is threaded into a neck vein (jugular vein) or thigh vein (femoral vein). Under X-ray guidance, it is passed through the larger blood vessels until it reaches the veins that drain the testicle. This catheter is about the size of a thin spaghetti noodle. The vein and its branches are identified by injecting them with a special X-ray contrast material (dye). Now that the target can be seen, the radiologist plugs the varicocele by passing small stainless steel coils through the catheter and releasing them into each branch of the varicocele. The coils stay in place, creating a blood clot that effectively blocks the vein. In addition to the small coils, an irritating liquid (such as a dense sugar solution) can be injected through the catheter. When the liquid hits the vein, it causes a scarring process to begin, which ultimately shuts off blood flow through the vein. Embolization can be done with very little recovery time. Men are often back to full activities within two days—shorter even than the healing time after microscopic or laparoscopic surgery.

A few years ago, we compared the success and cost of two different approaches: standard surgery and embolization. Both worked equally well and cost about the same, but embolization has the advantage of the shorter recovery period. Costs of these procedures vary widely at different centers across the United States.

As with any medical procedure, complications can happen no matter how skilled and careful the surgeon or radiologist. Fortunately, negative side effects are uncommon after either surgery or embolization to correct a varicocele. Perhaps the greatest risk, though it is just to be expected in some percentage of cases, is that the procedure may not improve a man's sperm quality. Sometimes the varicocele may not disappear after treatment. Usually this occurs because one of the tiny veins was missed, perhaps because it was positioned abnormally and could not be seen through the small incisions or on X rays done at the time of the procedure.

WHEN WILL YOU SEE RESULTS?

No matter how the varicocele is corrected, any improvements in sperm quality that result do not occur overnight. Since a complete cycle of sperm production takes about three months, it will take at least that long, and more likely six to nine months, to see measurable changes from eliminating the influence of the varicocele. So be patient! And if your sperm quality does not improve after varicocele correction, try not to get mired in regrets. Even the most expert infertility specialists have no crystal ball to predict future results when it comes to varicocele repair. All you can do is be a knowledgeable consumer and make what seems to be the most logical choice.

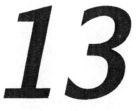

The Dry Ejaculation: Not a New Sexual Technique

Men sometimes experience an unexpected problem with ejaculation. Although they have all the feeling of orgasm, and can sense the muscles at the base of the penis tensing rhythmically, no semen spurts out. We call this a "dry ejaculation." It can be caused by several different kinds of medical problems. Although most men say that a dry ejaculation is still pleasurable, it obviously interferes with fertility and the cause of the problem needs to be identified.

WHAT HAPPENS DURING A DRY EJACULATION?

As we explained in chapter 6, ejaculation actually is a combination of three physical events. When sexual stimulation triggers the orgasm, a message flashes from the genital area through the nervous system to the brain and back again. A man actually feels the pleasure of orgasm because of these signals to his brain. Back down in the genital area, the *sympathetic nerves* direct the smooth muscle of the prostate and seminal vesicles to squeeze out the ingredients that make up the semen, protective fluid in which the sperm cells swim. Semen is mixed with sperm cells from the vas deferens and lower end of the epididymis. The fluid is released into the upper part of the urethra (urinary passageway). As the amount of fluid builds, it creates a pressure chamber between the bladder neck, which tightens down, and the external sphincter muscle, which closes off the urinary passageway. As ejaculation begins, another part of the nervous system takes over. The *somatic nerves* control skin sensations and the striated (striped) muscles that make the body move. During ejaculation, the striated muscles at the base of the penis squeeze and release about every second. With each contraction, the external sphincter opens and propels the semen out of the urethra in spurts.

Sometimes one element of ejaculation can be damaged, leaving the other parts of the process in working order. The most common cause of a dry ejaculation is that the bladder neck fails to close tightly. When ejaculation begins, the semen takes the path of least resistance, spurting backward into the bladder instead of out the tip of the penis. This is called retrograde ejaculation. This condition is not painful or harmful to a man's health. The semen simply mingles with a man's urine and will flow out the next time he urinates. Sometimes the semen makes the urine look cloudy. Microscopic examination of the urine after ejaculation will find sperm cells.

Another cause for dry ejaculation is that the sympathetic nerves that control the prostate and seminal vesicles do not fire up and semen never gathers in the upper urethra, as we discuss later in this chapter. A few men have dry ejaculations because their prostate and seminal vesicles have been removed as part of surgery for prostate or bladder cancer. These problems are discussed in the next chapter.

WHAT CAUSES RETROGRADE EJACULATION?

One of the common causes of retrograde ejaculation is damage to the bladder neck itself. When men have surgery to core out their enlarged prostate (often called a TURP, for *transurethral resection of the prostate*), or if a large, noncancerous prostate is "shelled out" through an open incision, the surgeon very commonly also removes some tissue from the bladder neck. Consequently, it does not shut tightly as orgasm approaches. Luckily, most men with enlarged prostates who need such surgery are older and not interested in having more children. Some men who have a TURP have no change in ejaculation, but there is no technique that reliably guarantees normal ejaculation after prostate surgery takes place. Newer, less-invasive methods of treating prostate enlargement, however, may minimize damage to the bladder neck and lessen the rate of retrograde ejaculation.

Another operation now rarely used, but common in the past, was performed to open up the bladder neck in young boys. Boys who had this surgery, called Y-V plasty because of the shape of the bladder neck incision, typically had problems with urination or had repeated urinary tract infections in childhood. Many of these young men grew up having retrograde ejaculation. It is difficult, though not impossible, to repair the bladder neck. Unfortunately, attempts to correct retrograde ejaculation can interfere with ease of urination.

Sometimes an injury to the urethra can result in a stricture, a tight band of scar tissue that interferes with the free flow of urine and semen (see chapter 6 for a description of the normal process of ejaculation). When the urethra is narrowed a man may have partial retrograde ejaculation. He may notice that semen does not spurt out at orgasm, but dribbles. Some semen may be forced backward into the bladder, as well.

> Brad had a nasty fall from his mountain bike when he hit an unexpected pothole. He landed with the bar of the bicycle right between his legs. He was in severe pain and went to the emergency room. His urine was bloody and his genital area was swollen. In the emergency room he had a test called a urethrogram, in which the doctor gently injected contrast dye into his urethra and took an X ray. A small tear was discovered in the urethra and a catheter was placed into Brad's bladder to allow it to heal. Brad's urination remained a bit slow, and he realized that the amount of semen he ejaculated was reduced. Several years later, Brad married and began to try to conceive a child with his wife. When they did not achieve pregnancy after a year, a semen analysis was done. The test revealed that Brad had a low normal sperm count with good motility, but a low volume of semen. Further tests revealed that he was ejaculating part of his semen back into his bladder because of scar tissue from his old injury. The scar tissue was opened and both urination and ejaculation returned to normal.

Retrograde ejaculation can also occur because of damage to the sympathetic nervous system. Young men who are diabetic can develop such damage, as can men with spinal cord injuries or multiple sclerosis. Occasionally, chemotherapy used to treat cancer can also damage these delicate nerves. Some surgical operations cut the pathways that send messages to the sympathetic nerves around the prostate. These surgeries include some operations that remove the rectum, either for inflammatory bowel disease or for rectal cancer. Another surgery that can injure the nerves is called a retroperitoneal lymph node dissection. This procedure is done in the course of treating some men who have testicular cancer (see the next chapter). Surgeons have recently developed techniques to try to avoid these nerves in many cases during rectal or node dissection surgery.

WHAT CAUSES COMPLETE PARALYSIS OF THE SYMPATHETIC NERVES?

Complete failure of the prostate, seminal vesicles, and vas deferens to squeeze out the semen and deposit it in the urethra is sometimes called *anejaculation,* or failure of emission (emission is a name for that part of the male orgasm). You cannot tell the difference between retrograde ejaculation and complete failure of emission by sensation. If you have dry ejaculations and no sperm cells are found in your urine, however, you have anejaculation. Most commonly, anejaculation happens when the sympathetic nerve pathways are severely damaged; for example, during rectal surgery or retroperitoneal node dissection surgery. When diseases, such as diabetes or multiple sclerosis, or injury to the spinal cord damages nerves severely, anejaculation can also result.

MEDICATIONS THAT SOMETIMES RESTORE EJACULATION

Some men can ejaculate semen normally again if they take medication that revs up the remaining intact sympathetic nerves around the prostate and seminal vesicles. Such drugs are called *sympathomimetics,* and you are probably familiar with some of them as over-the-counter or prescription-strength cold medications: pseudoephedrine hydrochloride (Sudafed), ephedrine sulfate (an ingredient in Marax), or phenylpropanolamine hydrochloride (Entex or Ornade, but each of these medications contains either an expectorant or an antihistamine, as well). As you might guess from their name, these medicines stimulate the sympathetic nerves. In the nose and throat, this reduces swelling in small blood vessels, allowing you to breathe more freely. Some of these drugs make your heart beat faster, increase your blood pressure, and give you the jitters. In a healthy man these side effects are generally not serious.

As part of their general stimulation of sympathetic nerves, sympath-omimetics tighten down the bladder neck and sometimes may increase the intensity of the contractions of the vas deferens and seminal vesicles during ejaculation.

In a man with dry ejaculation, sympathomimetics can sometimes restore the normal passage of semen through the urethra. Medication is more likely to work for retrograde ejaculation, however, than for complete failure of emission. If this type of medication fails, a few men may benefit from imipramine (Tofranil), which is usually used as an antidepressant. Unfortunately, after repeated doses, sympathomimetic medications can lose some or all of their effectiveness. To prevent such a loss, we generally recommend that a man only take the drug for the 10 days leading up to and around his partner's ovulation. Although some men wish there was a way to cure dry ejaculation just from a sexual standpoint, no medication is effective in the long term.

VIBRATORS ARE NOT JUST FOR FUN

At some time in your life, you may have tried a vibrator on yourself or your partner as a part of lovemaking. We think of vibrators as an aid to soothe sore muscles or as toys to enhance sexual pleasure, but in fact they can sometimes be a medical aid in infertility treatment. When men have spinal cord injuries and do not have normal sensation on their penis and scrotum, a vibrator can sometimes trigger an orgasm when other types of touch or mental sexual stimulation fail. The tiny nerves that sense vibration actually are separate from those that sense light touch. A vibrator produces a very strong, steady stimulation to these nerves.

The vibrators used in infertility treatment are "industrial strength," providing a higher intensity of vibration. They are typically placed directly under the head of the penis or are moved around the ridge that rings the head of the penis (coronal ridge) until the most effective spot is found. Sometimes a gentler, commercially available vibrator will also do the trick.

Some men who have injuries to the upper part of the spinal cord (i.e., they are paralyzed from the neck down) are at risk for a possibly life-threatening medical problem called *autonomic dysreflexia*, which is brought on by intense stimulation such as that produced by the vibrator. Because the spinal cord no longer controls the sympathetic nervous system effectively, various strong sensations such as those provoked by a vibrator are accompanied by severe headaches, high blood pressure, and sweating. A man with a spinal cord injury should not experiment with a vibrator at home until he has discussed it with his physician, or tried it in a medical setting where emergency care can be given. Certain medications can also prevent, or at least minimize, autonomic dysreflexia. If a man proves not to be at risk for this reaction, then he can try a vibrator at home. Ejaculating more regularly may sometimes improve sperm counts and motility in a man who has a spinal cord injury.

USING ELECTRICITY
TO EJACULATE

Another way to trigger ejaculation of semen in a man with failure of emission is to use electrical stimulation (electroejaculation). A probe about an inch in diameter is placed in the patient's rectum. A gradually increasing electrical impulse stimulates the nerves around the prostate and seminal vesicles, causing ejaculation of semen. This type of ejaculation does not involve a pleasurable orgasm, however. In fact, it is quite a painful sensation. Men who have spinal cord injuries with a loss of sensation in the rectal and genital area can undergo electroejaculation as an office procedure while they are awake (although again, some patients risk autonomic dysreflexia, and protective measures should be taken). Other men with normal sensation need to be put under a general or spinal anesthetic for this procedure. Perhaps in a few years, more selective nerve stimulators will be developed that do not produce such a painful sensation.

In the meanwhile, however, electroejaculation is successful in about three-quarters of men in whom it is tried. The sperm counts are usually good, but the motility is poor. Nonetheless, the washed sperm can be used with intrauterine insemination (IUI). Even if the quality is poor and IUI fails, the semen almost always contains live sperm cells useful for in vitro fertilization with intracytoplasmic sperm injection, or IVF-ICSI (see chapter 16).

Either vibration stimulation or electroejaculation may result in retrograde ejaculation. In that case, the sperm cells must be separated from the urine by using some special washing techniques. Electroejaculation or stimulation with a vibrator can be repeated, if necessary, without damaging the reproductive system.

RETRIEVING SPERM CELLS
FROM A MAN'S URINE

When medication does not correct retrograde ejaculation, or if electroejaculation or vibrator stimulation produces retrograde ejaculation, sperm cells can be retrieved from a man's urine just after he ejaculates. This process is not particularly difficult, but instructions for collection should be very specific and followed to the letter. Urine is typically quite acid and will kill sperm cells almost on contact. Semen, in contrast to urine, is an alkaline fluid. If you ever took Basic Chemistry 101, you may recall that water is neutral and has a pH level of 7. Acidic liquids have pH values less than 7, and alkaline solutions have a pH between 7 and 14.

In order to make urine a little more hospitable to sperm, it needs to be made less acid. This is usually done pretty easily by having a man take sodium bicarbonate tablets or powder the day before, and the day of, his sperm retrieval. He must also avoid any acid-producing foods and drinks for those two days. When he comes to the doctor's office, he gives a urine sample, and its pH is measured. If the urine is alkaline, the man ejaculates, either through his own self-stimulation or with vibratory or electrical assistance. Once ejaculation has taken place, he urinates again into a collection cup or a small catheter can be placed to drain his bladder.

This fluid, which should contain urine mixed with sperm, is sent immediately to the laboratory. There the sperm are washed out of the urine and *resuspended,* that is, put into a nutrient liquid. The sample can be used for IUI or IVF-ICSI.

SURGICAL SPERM ASPIRATION

If none of the methods described in this chapter result in obtaining live sperm cells, a minor outpatient surgery may be necessary. Under local anesthetic, the surgeon makes a very small incision in the scrotal skin, allowing him to get to one of the vas deferens. Remember that this is the tube that carries ripe sperm cells from the epididymis (see chapter 4). A small incision is made in the vas deferens to partially open it. The surgeon squeezes the vas deferens and collects the fluid and sperm cells that ooze out of the opening created (called a "partial vasotomy"). Then the opening is sewed shut with a few tiny sutures, and the skin is also closed. The sperm cells can be used that day for IUI or IVF-ICSI, or frozen for the future.

Some infertility specialists have tried to obtain sperm cells by inserting a needle into the vas deferens or epididymis and drawing out sperm cells and fluid. These techniques can create scarring, however, making it hard to repeat them more than once or twice. The amount of sperm cells obtained is also not typically as good as with the partial vasotomy or open aspiration from the epididymis. Recovering from a vasotomy just involves some local soreness, similar or less severe than a one-sided vasectomy.

14

Adding
Insult to Injury:
Infertility after
Cancer Treatment

Advances in cancer treatment for a number of malignancies of child-hood and young adulthood leave many young men with good life expectancies. Testicular cancer, the most common tumor in young men, has a five-year survival rate (the statistic used to indicate that someone has probably beaten cancer), of 95 percent according to the *1998 Cancer Facts and Figures,* published by the American Cancer Society. Hodgkin's disease, a cancer of the lymph nodes and immune system seen in young people, now has a five-year survival rate of 81 percent. The death rate for all childhood cancers has decreased by 57 percent since the early 1970s, so that today, 72 percent of children diagnosed with cancer live for at least five years.

Unfortunately, our ability to control cancer and extend life still comes at the price of treatment side effects that may reduce the quality of that life. One of the frequent ill effects of successful cancer treatment is male infertility.

DOES THE CANCER ITSELF
CAUSE INFERTILITY?

A few types of cancer have a specific link to male infertility. These malignancies are more common in men whose fertility was damaged by a genetic or developmental problem. For example, men whose testicles did not descend normally, but had to be brought down to the scrotum with surgery, have an increased risk for testicular cancer. Although most men who develop testicular cancer had normal fertility before their diagnosis, a small percentage of these tumors occur in men whose testicles have never been healthy sperm producers.

Some types of cancer also produce fevers or abnormal hormones that can temporarily interfere with sperm production until cancer treatment corrects the situation. These include leukemia, lymphoma, Hodgkin's disease, and testicular cancer. The trauma to the body from anesthesia and surgery performed to diagnose or treat the cancer can also lower sperm counts in the short term. The severe and more long-term infertility seen in cancer survivors, however, is usually related to chemotherapy drugs or radiation therapy used to treat the cancer.

WHY CANCER TREATMENT
CAUSES INFERTILITY

Radiation or chemotherapy kills tumors by damaging them while they are busy growing. Once you become an adult, most cells in your body stop reproducing themselves, or at least do so very slowly. There are a few exceptions, including your hair, blood and immune system cells, sperm cells, and cells that become cancerous. These cells grow and divide rapidly. A cell that is resting may get damaged by radiation or toxic chemotherapy drugs, but can often repair itself. A cell that is in the midst of copying its genetic material and dividing into two new cells is much more fragile. Cancer treatments capitalize on this fact, using toxic chemicals or radiation to kill all or most cancer cells without killing the normal cells around them. Since cancer treatments target rapidly dividing cells, they can often cause a man to lose his hair, become anemic, have low resistance to disease, or stop producing sperm cells.

The parent spermatogonia that produce all immature sperm cells (see chapter 4) have a fairly good ability to resist radiation or chemotherapy damage. The sperm cells that are in the ripening stages, however, are very easily damaged. If some parent cells remain intact after cancer treatment, sperm production can eventually resume (though perhaps not at the same level as before). If the treatment is so harsh that all the parent cells are killed, however, permanent infertility can occur.

THE IMPACT OF RADIATION

Radiation treatment is aimed at the area where the tumor cells are. If radiation is aimed at the upper body—for example, the "mantle fields" covering the shoulders and parts of the chest sometimes used for Hodgkin's disease—the testicles may not get much exposure to the harmful rays. If radiation is aimed at the groin—for example, to treat a kind of testicular cancer called seminoma—the remaining healthy testicle, even if protected by a special shield, may get a big dose, too. The higher the dose of radiation to the testicles, the more damage to sperm production. It takes only a dose of 6 gray (gray, abbreviated as Gy, are the units used to measure radiation) to the testicles to permanently stop sperm cell production. In contrast, it may take anywhere from 2.5 to 7 Gy to kill a tumor.

Luckily, the testicles can be at least partially protected with lead shields from radiation delivered to the pelvic area. Some radiation still gets to the testicles from scatter inside the body, however. The beam aimed at a nearby organ bounces off, and some radiation ricochets into the testicular tissue. Occasionally, radiation needs to be aimed directly at a testicle; for example, when leukemia cells are located there. When a dose of radiation is given to a man's whole body to kill a maximum number of tumor cells in preparation for a bone marrow transplant, the dose to the testicles is usually so high that fertility does not recover.

When a man has a tumor in his brain, radiation used to treat it may sometimes damage the areas that produce messenger hormones involved in controlling the testicle's production of sperm cells. Missing hormones can sometimes be replaced, jump-starting fertility again. Sometimes it is not enough to simply inject the hormones into a man's bloodstream once a day or several times a week. He may need to wear a small pump system to deliver the hormone into his circulation in a dosage pattern that mimics the timing and amounts of hormone that his brain or pituitary gland would normally produce.

THE IMPACT OF CHEMOTHERAPY
ON MEN'S FERTILITY

Not that much is known about the damage to male fertility caused by individual chemotherapy drugs or the combinations used to treat various cancers. It is clear that both the type and the total dosage of drugs used to treat the cancer are factors in whether sperm production will be decreased. Age matters, too. When a boy is below the age of puberty during his chemotherapy, his testicles may be somewhat more resistant to damage. On the other hand, men over age 40 have poorer recovery of fertility after chemotherapy. Recovery of sperm production often takes one to four years after chemotherapy has ended. After four years, fertility is unlikely to improve more.

The chemotherapy drugs most damaging to the sperm-producing cells in the testicles are called *alkylating drugs.* They include cyclophosphamide, chlorambucil, busulfan, procarbazine, nitrosoureas, nitrogen mustard, and l-phenylalanine mustard. These particular drugs have often been used as part of the treatment for lymphomas or Hodgkin's disease. Men with testicular cancer do not usually receive alkylating drugs. At least half of the men recover some sperm production after combination chemotherapy for testicular cancer that includes the drugs VP-16, cis-platinum, or bleomycin. Cis-platinum, however, also is known to permanently damage sperm production at high doses. A combination of chemotherapy and radiation therapy also may be more damaging to fertility than either one given alone.

Because the testicles appear to be more resistant to chemotherapy damage before puberty, researchers have tried giving men hormones to stop sperm cell production during chemotherapy in the hopes that fertility would be more likely to return after cancer treatment. Unfortunately, none of the protective hormone treatments has worked, so far.

FERTILITY AFTER
BONE MARROW TRANSPLANT

When a man needs a bone marrow transplant, he is first given a very strong dose of radiation to his whole body, or an extremely harsh dose and combination of chemotherapy drugs (or sometimes both radiation and chemotherapy). These treatments are designed to kill all cancer cells in his body, including those in the blood and lymph circulation systems. These treatments are so strong, however, that his own bone marrow, which produces his blood cells, is killed off. After the cancer treatment, his bone marrow will be replaced either with marrow cells collected from his own body beforehand, or, if there is a chance that his own stored marrow would contain cancer cells, with marrow from a matched donor.

Recovery of sperm production after a bone marrow transplant occurs, but only rarely. If sperm cells are found in a man's semen again after bone marrow transplantation from a donor, they are genetically his own, and not his bone marrow donor's cells. These sperm cells would be produced by the man's own parent cells that had survived through his cancer treatment. It is only his blood cells that are replaced by the donor's cells.

When Mickey was informed that he needed a bone marrow transplant to treat his leukemia, he and his wife Tina were newly married and had not yet begun to try for a pregnancy. The oncologist sat them both down in her office and said the procedure would end Mickey's fertility permanently. She offered sperm banking to the couple and they accepted. When Mickey had survived for two years without a leukemia recurrence, Tina was inseminated with his stored semen and quickly conceived. Their son was born nine months later, with all his fingers and toes, as well as a raging appetite! He was such an active and demanding toddler that Tina was not too worried about whether enough semen remained to conceive a second child.

When the little boy was about two, Tina went through several weeks of nausea and fatigue. She could not figure out what was wrong, and went to her family doctor. She and Mickey were both shocked to find that she was pregnant. They made an appointment to see Mickey's oncologist, frightened about the possibility that a child born after cancer treatment might not be healthy. The oncologist again took both spouses into her office and turned to Tina. "Are you sure your husband fathered this pregnancy?" she asked abruptly. Tina was so angry that she could not even answer for a moment. Mickey said later that if the physician had been male, he would have punched his lights out. The oncologist went on to say that she had never heard of a case of a man fathering a child after a bone marrow transplant. Tina later found out from an oncology nurse who had befriended the couple during treatment that a number of cases like theirs had been reported in the medical literature. The couple waited until they had cooled off, and then wrote a letter to the oncologist, suggesting she use more sensitivity the next time she had a similar situation in her office. They ended up seeing a geneticist who reassured them about the probable health of their baby, and indeed, their daughter was just as healthy as their first child, although luckily born with an easier temperament.

WHEN CANCER SURGERY REMOVES
PART OF THE REPRODUCTIVE SYSTEM

Treating cancer sometimes involves an operation that removes part of the reproductive system, including the testicles, or the prostate and seminal vesicles. Testicular cancer rarely involves both testicles, so even though one must be removed to contain the cancer, the remaining testicle is available to produce sperm, as long as it was working well before cancer treatment and is not too badly damaged by radiation or chemotherapy. One healthy testicle can maintain a normal sperm count.

When surgery is used to treat cancer of the bladder or prostate, the vas deferens, prostate, and seminal vesicles are part of the area removed. Thus, a man continues to make sperm cells, but they remain trapped in the testicles. Although a man can still experience the sensation of orgasm when he has the right kind of sexual stimulation, he produces no seminal fluid, so nothing flows out of his penis.

Most men with prostate or bladder cancer are over age 50 and have finished their families. Occasionally, however, a younger man will have cancer, or a man in his 50s, 60s, or even 70s would still like to father a child. As chapter 16 explains, minor surgery could be used to retrieve sperm cells from a man's epididymis or testicle. In vitro fertilization with intracytoplasmic sperm injection (IVF-ICSI) would then be necessary to achieve a pregnancy.

AVOIDING INFERTILITY
AFTER TESTICULAR CANCER

Young men who have testicular cancer sometimes have a surgery called *retroperitoneal lymph node dissection*. During this operation, the surgeon removes a chain of lymph nodes that receives drainage from the testicles. When testicular cancer spreads, it often does so through this lymph drainage system. When nodes are positive (i.e., contain cancer cells), chemotherapy is usually needed as part of the cancer treatment. A node dissection may also be done after chemotherapy to remove scar tissue or remaining questionable areas that could contain active cancer.

Node dissections can injure the nerves that control ejaculation of semen, causing dry ejaculation (see chapter 13). Surgeons have changed the way they do nerve dissections to try to spare these important nerves. Most men recover normal ejaculation of semen after nerve-sparing surgery, but some may continue to have dry ejaculations.

When the tumor in the testicle is found at an early stage, doctors will sometimes avoid performing a node dissection surgery, instead recommending surveillance—a program of watchful waiting to see if the cancer will reappear in the body. Men on surveillance must be prepared for frequent doctor visits and repeated medical tests. If they skip a follow-up appointment, they could be putting their lives at risk.

THE HEALTH OF CHILDREN
BORN AFTER A MAN'S EXPOSURE
TO RADIATION OR CHEMOTHERAPY

Several follow-up studies have looked at rates of birth defects in children born to cancer survivors after their treatment. Thus far, there is no evidence that children born after a father's chemotherapy or radiation therapy have a higher rate of birth defects or health problems. There have even been a few babies conceived during chemotherapy or radiation therapy, before the man's sperm counts decreased too much. Although sperm cells could theoretically be genetically damaged by these cancer treatments, no evidence of genetic damage was seen in the children.

Although these studies are reassuring, the number of babies studied has only been a few thousand. With a larger group of children, some small increases in health problems could become apparent. Thus, men are counseled to bank their sperm cells (see below) before cancer treatment, and to use contraception during chemotherapy or radiation therapy, as well as for three to six months afterward. By that time, any sperm cells directly exposed to cancer treatment should be used up. Some experts believe men should wait up to two years after radiation therapy or chemotherapy to father a child. Not only do most recurrences of cancer occur during the first two years after treatment, but the extra time may allow the body to repair some of the genetic damage that could theoretically affect sperm cells.

Children born to cancer survivors do not have unusual rates of cancer themselves. A few types of cancer may have a genetic basis, and run in families. These sometimes, but not always, include the childhood cancer retinoblastoma; cancer of the breast, ovary, or colon that occurs at an unusually young age; or a minority of testicular tumors or cases of Hodgkin's disease. If your family tree includes an unusually strong pattern of cancer, or several relatives on one side with a similar type of cancer or cancer at an unusually young age, you may wish to have genetic counseling (see chapter 7) as part of your decision process about having children.

THE IMPORTANCE OF BANKING SPERM BEFORE CANCER TREATMENT

Until recently, many physicians did not advise men to bank sperm (i.e., freeze samples of semen for future creation of a pregnancy) before cancer treatment. Many men did not meet criteria for sperm banking at the time of cancer diagnosis because their disease or diagnostic procedures had already resulted in depressed sperm counts and motility. Physicians reasoned that sperm of lower quality would not freeze and thaw well. Insemination with such thawed semen was unlikely to result in a pregnancy, so that the expense and trouble of sperm banking would be wasted. With the advent of IVF-ICSI, however, it became clear that you only need a few live sperm cells to produce healthy pregnancies. Now most cancer centers suggest sperm banking for any man who is going to have chemotherapy, or radiation therapy or surgery in the pelvic area, and would like to keep the option to have children. Sperm banking can also be used successfully with young teenagers. Sperm banking would only be of no use if there were no live sperm cells in a man's semen.

Another objection to sperm banking was that it could delay treatment, especially with very aggressive cancers like acute leukemia or advanced testicular cancer. A study at our own institution, the Cleveland Clinic Foundation, showed that men about to start cancer treatment could collect a useful amount of semen in less than a week by shortening the usual time interval between semen samples. Although it is always preferable to collect sperm cells that have not been exposed to radiation or chemotherapy drugs, you also have the option to store some sperm during the first few days of cancer treatment. If you conceive a pregnancy using that sample, you may want to have genetic counseling and consider prenatal diagnosis to determine if the fetus has suffered any genetic damage.

In the near future, it may be possible to use a needle or minor surgery to locate and extract some parent spermatogonia from a man's testicle before cancer treatment, freeze the parent cells, and later thaw and transplant them back into his testicle, where they should resume producing new sperm cells. This procedure is already possible in animals, but has not yet been used successfully in humans.

The costs of banking sperm may be partially or wholly covered by your insurance. Most sperm banks charge between $600 and $2,000 for processing and storing the semen samples for five years. Since cancer is a life-threatening disease, we recommend that you decide what you would want to happen to your banked sperm if you died. Some men would want their banked samples destroyed, especially since most sperm banks charge a yearly storage fee to keep the samples. If you are married, you and your wife may agree that she should have the right to use your stored semen to conceive a pregnancy even if you were no longer alive. Some parents of young men who died without having children have requested a court order to use stored sperm to get a surrogate mother pregnant. Then the parents would raise their own grandchild. Unless you specify your wishes for your stored semen in a written and signed document called an *advance directive,* the courts will have the right to decide on the fate of your sperm samples. Even with an advance directive, your family might have to take legal action to follow your wishes, but they would have a better chance of getting the court to rule in their favor.

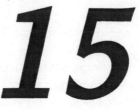

Does Lifestyle Contribute to Male Infertility?

Men often wonder if there is something about their occupation or health habits that is affecting their fertility. If so, perhaps it is something that could be changed. Although there are only a few lifestyle factors that clearly disrupt men's fertility, a variety of health habits or activities appear to have a small impact on semen quality. If a man's sperm count and motility were terrific, these factors might not affect his ability to start a pregnancy. If his semen quality is borderline, however, each change he makes toward better health may be the one that makes the difference in conception. If you make some healthy changes, give them time to work. Remember that your sperm production needs a three-month lead time to start to show improvement.

DR. THOMAS'S HEALTHY-SPERM DIET

Uh, oh, are we going to offer you a plan to eat yourself into fertility? Don't worry. Although we would love to publish a surefire way to improve your semen quality through nutrition, we are too responsible to make such claims. There is no one nutrient or food that has been scientifically proved to enhance men's fertility. As we noted in past chapters, however, nutrition may have some impact. Men who are very obese or emaciated may have abnormal hormone levels, which in turn affect sperm production. Antioxidant vitamins, particularly A, C, and E, may also have some impact on semen quality. Experts often recommend getting a good dose of vitamins from your daily diet, since your body may absorb the vitamins more efficiently from food than from supplement pills. Vitamin A includes the carotenoid chemicals found not only in carrots, but other yellow, orange, or red fruits and vegetables such as sweet potatoes, pumpkins, red peppers, and dried peaches. Spinach is also an excellent source. Foods rich in vitamin C include citrus fruits (oranges, grapefruit, papayas, lemons, limes), as well as green vegetables such as broccoli or brussels sprouts. Vitamin E (the tocopherols) is found in high levels in fortified dry cereals, cooked multigrain cereals, wheat germ, shrimp, almonds, filberts, and sunflower seeds.

You can also take vitamin supplements, but make sure not to take a higher dose than the daily recommended allowance, unless your physician specifically instructs you to do so. In fact, we do not suggest that you take any vitamin supplement until you discuss it with your doctor. Even the recommended daily dose of vitamin E can cause excessive bleeding if a man is also taking high doses of aspirin, other anti-inflammatory drugs, or is on anticoagulant medications such as coumadin. If you are in good health and not taking any prescription medication, it is usually safe to take a good-quality multivitamin that contains vitamins A and C, as well as recommended daily doses of magnesium and zinc, chemicals that may be important in the prostate. You can also take a total of 400 international units (IUs) a day of vitamin E.

With all the evidence that a low-fat diet helps to prevent heart disease and some types of cancer, it is just common sense to limit your fat intake. A good strategy is to follow the advice of the American Cancer Society and eat five servings of fruits or vegetables a day (and leave that cheese sauce off your cauliflower).

DOES PHYSICAL FITNESS LEAD TO REPRODUCTIVE FITNESS?

There is no direct proof that increasing your physical fitness will improve your semen quality, but again, within limits it certainly will not hurt. Men who are extreme athletes—those who run over 100 miles a week or bicycle more than 50 miles a week—may actually have some decrease in sperm counts and motility. Perhaps their percentage of body fat drops to a level that alters their hormone balance. On the other hand, men who train to good, but not superb, levels of endurance appear to have increased testosterone levels. This, in turn, might enhance sex drive or improve the environment for sperm cell production.

THE BOXER SHORTS
VERSUS BRIEFS CONTROVERSY

Since we know that the testicles produce healthy sperm when their temperature is slightly below body temperature, some infertility specialists have worried that wearing athletic briefs would heat up the testicles and interfere with semen quality. They recommended for years that men wear boxer shorts to give their testicles a nice cool breeze. More recently, studies have shown that, at least in men with normal sperm counts, there is no advantage to semen quality of wearing boxer shorts instead of knitted briefs.

One well-known urologist even went a step further, helping to develop a special "testicular cooling device," a jockstrap containing a water-cooled, mini air conditioner for the testicles. A man was instructed not only to wear this device under his clothes in the daytime, but also to sleep with his genitals uncovered, his legs apart, and his head slightly lower than his feet in order to keep blood from flowing back in the veins of the scrotum. Although early results were somewhat promising, men with infertility will be relieved to know that this program has not won general acceptance as a treatment.

HOT TUBS ARE NOT SO HOT FOR SPERM!

Even if chilling the family jewels is not likely to help your sperm count, boiling them could still be a mistake. Another factor not scientifically proven to affect fertility, but possibly a problem, is the practice of soaking in hot tubs. Again, for the man with borderline semen quality, the exposure to water hotter than body temperature could potentially damage sperm cell production to a point that pregnancy would be less likely to occur. Even a high fever during a viral illness can sometimes temporarily damage your semen quality. Some studies have actually shown that frequent use of a sauna can depress sperm counts temporarily. Our advice is, if you are trying for a pregnancy, skip the sauna and hightail it out of the hot tub.

SMOKING IS NOT GOOD FOR SPERM (OR ANY OTHER PART OF YOUR BODY)

Although smoking has not been proven to reduce male fertility in general, several research studies have shown that men who smoke have somewhat lower sperm counts, and motility, and more abnormally shaped sperm cells. It is easier to see these changes in groups of healthy men than in men who come to infertility clinics, since many in this latter group have other medical causes for their poor semen quality. Although it is hard to prove that smokers as a group have reduced fertility, men whose semen quality is already somewhat low may benefit from quitting use of tobacco products, including cigarettes, cigars, or chewing tobacco. Several studies have found that quitting smoking can improve semen quality.

Often in marriages, both partners smoke. It is very clear that smoking interferes with women's fertility and increases the risk of miscarriage. If your wife smokes, why not try quitting together as part of your effort to have a baby? Not only is it a positive factor in your fertility, but it is probably the one best change you can make for your future health and long life.

ALCOHOL AND MALE FERTILITY

Alcohol is another of those factors that may be the straw that breaks the camel's back for men with borderline fertility. It is clear that men who are very heavy drinkers can damage their fertility over years of alcohol abuse. When alcohol damages the liver, the hormone balance in the reproductive system is also affected. Alcohol has also been shown to have direct toxic effects on the tissue of the testicles. For men who drink moderately, most studies have not shown a link with fertility, although daily drinkers in one study had a higher percentage of abnormal sperm cells. Again, if you are trying for a pregnancy, it is simple common sense to reduce your alcohol to a level that seems unlikely to interfere, perhaps a unit a day at most, with a unit meaning one 6-ounce glass of wine, one 12-ounce can of regular beer (not malt ale), or one shot of hard liquor.

Again, if your partner is a heavy drinker, helping her to cut down is even more crucial before you try to have a baby. Alcohol use during pregnancy has clearly been linked to the fetal alcohol syndrome, which causes physical birth defects and learning disabilities. Even moderate levels of alcohol use during pregnancy can be dangerous, and pregnant women are advised not to drink alcohol at all.

DO I HAVE TO
GIVE UP COFFEE, TOO?

In women, coffee drinking has recently been linked to trouble getting pregnant. Heavy coffee consumption has also been related to male infertility in one Italian study (lots of caffeine in that espresso!). It is unlikely that drinking a cup of coffee a day will affect your chances of conceiving, but this is another area where heavy users could possibly benefit from decreasing. Recent research also has shown that caffeine has some addictive qualities, so do not be surprised if cutting down on coffee temporarily gives you headaches or makes you irritable. It still could be worthwhile.

RECREATIONAL DRUGS
AND MALE FERTILITY

Although some studies have suggested that regular marijuana use damages semen quality, the evidence is controversial. We know that men who become addicted to drugs in the opiate family—cocaine, crack cocaine, or heroin—eventually lose their desire for sex and have trouble getting erections. The hormonal impacts of these drugs may also reduce sperm counts and motility, but it is hard to find research showing these effects in humans. In rats, it was recently shown that daily doses of cocaine equivalent to those taken by a heavy human user produced direct damage to the sperm-producing tissue in the testicle.

We would counsel any man trying to conceive a pregnancy with his partner to stop using all recreational drugs. In fact, we would give him the same advice even if he were not trying to conceive!

USING ANABOLIC STEROIDS
FOR ATHLETICS

Anabolic steroids are chemical substances that some men and women use (or misuse) to enhance their athletic performance, be it for strength or speed. The term "anabolic" means that these hormones help the human body to build up muscle mass.

Anabolic steroids are very similar chemically to the hormone testosterone. Scientists created these new drugs by chemically altering testosterone in ways that prolong its effect. Anabolic steroids have a few medically approved uses. They are sometimes given to patients who have diseases that cause weakness and wasting—for example, AIDS or advanced cancer. In these situations, the steroids may restore a patient's appetite for food, muscle strength, and vitality. Athletes have used anabolic steroids against the advice of most medical experts. Combined with exercise and a high-protein diet, anabolic steroids do increase muscle mass and strength. Unfortunately, these same athletes who work so hard at developing their bodies for a particular sport may suffer significant health problems in return for the edge steroids offer.

As we saw in chapter 4, testosterone is manufactured by the Leydig cells of the testicles. Only a small amount (about 6 to 7 milligrams) is made each day. This is sufficient for normal sexual function and sperm cell production. When a man is given extra testosterone, it suppresses sperm manufacture. In fact, high doses of testosterone were considered for use as a male contraceptive, although other hormone side effects halted this line of research.

Anabolic steroids act like testosterone. Most athletes who use steroids take extremely high doses, far beyond the hormone levels that a man's body would normally produce. Athletes often add one type of anabolic steroid to another (called "stacking") and take them for periods of six to twelve weeks (called "cycles"). After a cycle, the athlete often takes a break for three to six months, presumably to get his body functions to return to normal. In many cases, however, this period is not long enough for all the effects of the anabolic steroids to disappear.

While a man is on steroids, his sperm cell production decreases, sometimes shutting off completely. After several weeks, his testicles actually may shrink visibly in size and become softer. Perhaps that is why some body builders can fit into those tiny bathing suits! Some men may also develop high blood pressure, male pattern baldness, breast enlargement, liver disease, acne, or elevated cholesterol levels. Women athletes using anabolic steroids also may grow increased facial hair, develop deeper voices, have the clitoris enlarge, or stop having menstrual cycles. Some men and women become unusually aggressive, a condition often termed "steroid rage." Men often say their sex drive is quite high on anabolic steroids.

When an athlete stops taking steroids, it may require a minimum of six months for body systems, including sperm cell production, to return to normal. We have recently seen patients who took a year to regain normal semen quality.

Some anabolic steroids are taken by mouth. Others are injected into the arm or hip muscle. Almost all of these drugs are acquired on the black market, so their purity and overall safety is never assured. Perhaps one of the most dangerous aspects of using steroids is that men who work out together often share their hormone-injecting needles. You may think your buddy at the gym is a clean-living guy, but what if he has HIV or hepatitis? These diseases not only threaten a man's health, but can be sexually transmitted to his partner.

Do not confuse anabolic steroids with another type of steroid called "corticosteroids." This group of drugs, including prednisone, cortisone, or Medrol, is prescribed to treat intense allergic reactions, severe inflammation, or to prevent rejection of a transplanted organ. These medications are not used for bodybuilding or athletics.

PRESCRIPTION DRUGS
AND MALE INFERTILITY

Although we think of medications prescribed by a doctor as contributing to our health, some can also have negative effects on sperm production or function. The physician who wrote the prescription may not always be aware of these side effects, or even that you are trying to conceive a pregnancy. Thus, you should always tell your infertility specialist about any prescription medications you are taking. We have mentioned the impact of chemotherapy for cancer and drugs that interfere with hormones in other chapters. Here we would like to mention the generic and trade names of some medications that can damage sperm cell production: ketoconazole (Nizoral), which is used to treat fungal infections; sulfasalazine (Azulfidine), often used by people who have ulcerative colitis; valproic acid (Depakene), a medicine used to prevent seizures; spironolactone (Aldactone, Aldactazide), used as a diuretic for people with hypertension or liver or heart failure; and allopurinol (Zyloprim), a medication used to reduce the high levels of uric acid that produce gout.

Some medications also damage the sperm cells' ability to fertilize the oocyte. These include calcium channel blockers, a group of medications used to treat hypertension and heart disease and including commonly prescribed drugs such as nifedipine (Procardia, Adalat) and verapamil (Calan, Verelan, Isoptin). Fertilization can also be affected by colcichine (Colbenamid), prescribed for gouty arthritis; nitrofurantoin (Macrobid), an antibiotic often used to treat urinary tract infections; and minocycline (Minocin, Dynacin), an antibiotic used to treat a variety of infections by gram-negative bacteria.

EMOTIONAL STRESS AND INFERTILITY

Stress has become a byword in folk wisdom about infertility. "You're trying too hard," couples are told, "go on a vacation!" Theoretically, stress could impact a man's fertility by altering the hormones produced in his brain and pituitary gland. A change in the messenger hormones could then slow down sperm production in the testicles. The kind of stress producing such a change would have to be pretty major. One recent study measured job stress and stressful life events in healthy men who agreed to give a semen sample. Despite the researchers' using some very fancy computerized semen analyses, only one type of stressor had a mild effect on sperm motility—the recent death of a close family member.

Two other studies have looked at the stress of in vitro fertilization (IVF) itself, comparing semen quality from a sample men provided when they first entered a fertility program to that of the sample they gave when the pressure was really on—the day of egg retrieval. In the meanwhile, enough time had passed that the anxiety of going through IVF could have had an impact on sperm cell production. In both studies, very few of the men had abnormal semen analyses at the beginning. In one study, no overall changes were seen when the two semen samples were compared. In the second study, 11 percent of men had normal semen analyses the first time, but abnormal ones on the day of egg retrieval. Again, if psychological stress plays a role, it appears to be a rather mild one.

PHYSICAL STRESS

A variety of physical stressors can interfere with sperm cell production—for example, a high fever, a severe infection, or an acute or chronic illness. Exposure to toxic chemicals or to radiation is also an important physical stressor. After an unusual medical or physical stress, recovery of normal sperm cell production can take from three to six months.

CAN YOUR JOB MAKE YOU INFERTILE?

Some occupations expose men to chemicals known to endanger fertility, such as pesticides (DDT, chlordecone), lead, mercury vapor, carbon disulfide, dibromochloropropane (an ingredient in pesticides), carbaryl (a pesticide), ethylene dibromide (used in fumigation), sterene and acetone (used in making plastics), or ethylene glycol ethers (used in paints, inks, and paint thinners). Some men also work around military radar, are exposed to microwaves on the job, or are exposed accidentally to excess levels of radiation on the job. These exposures can damage sperm cell production. Even a work environment that is unusually hot, such as a ceramics plant or a steel mill, may alter semen quality. Welders have also been shown to have a higher rate of some semen abnormalities, perhaps due to exposure to heat, chromium, or toxic vapors. Even driving a vehicle for a living has been suspected to reduce semen quality in some men.

If you believe your job may be affecting your fertility, you have a right to ask for a change in your working conditions. Your infertility specialist may be able to help by writing a letter to your employer explaining the problem.

POLLUTANTS IN THE ENVIRONMENT
AND MALE FERTILITY

As we have mentioned earlier in this book, controversy still exists on whether men's sperm counts are declining in the industrialized part of the world. Statistics for the United States have been interpreted recently as showing a real decline in semen quality for the years 1940 through 1990. A study of Canadian fertility clinics showed a similar trend for 1984 to 1996. Other European countries, including France, Belgium,

Scotland, and England, have reported declines, while Finland has not. It is interesting that Finland has also escaped the rising rates of testicular cancer seen in many other countries, including the other Scandinavian nations.

One theory is that this decrease in male fertility, if genuine, is related to increased levels of environmental pollutants that have estrogenlike effects in the human body. Such pollutants have been linked to fertility problems in wildlife. So far, this is just a theory for humans, however. Another suggestion is that a mother's smoking during her pregnancy could affect her son's fertility. Finland had low rates of women smokers during the period studied. As we have seen in earlier sections of this chapter, a wide variety of poor health habits common in industrial countries could potentially have some effect on men's semen quality. A growing rate of urethritis related to sexually transmitted bacteria could also play a role.

To complicate matters even more, not all estrogenlike chemicals are bad for men. Plants manufacture chemicals called phytoestrogens, such as lignans and isoflavonoids. These chemicals may prevent some types of cancer, and are common in Asian diets based on soy products. They are also found in whole-grain cereals, seeds, and some berries. Phytoestrogens are not known to have any ill effects on human fertility.

GETTING HEALTHY

If there is an area within your health habits that could be improved—whether it be better nutrition, more regular exercise, quitting tobacco or recreational drugs, cutting down on alcohol and coffee, avoiding exposure to heat and toxic chemicals—now is the time to make some changes. It is a lot more painless to live a healthier lifestyle than to spend thousands of dollars on diagnosing and treating infertility, especially if your semen quality is only mildly low. Furthermore, infertility treatments will just bring you needle pricks, uncomfortable exams, and irritability, whereas being more fit and healthy will not only make you feel good, but should have positive impacts on your partner and your future children.

> Brian worked as an assembler in an engine factory. His wife, Maureen, was a secretary. Their favorite time was the summer, when they could take their large motorboat out on the lake on weekends. After three years of marriage they felt ready to start a

family, but after two more years, no pregnancy had occurred. They went through a pretty thorough infertility evaluation, but little was found wrong on either side. Brian's semen had a low percentage of normal sperm cells, and he had an excess of white cells in his semen that did not clear up with antibiotics. Three cycles of intrauterine insemination also did not result in conception. The specialists told them they could try IVF, since that was the most effective treatment for infertility with unclear cause. They also pointed out, however, that both spouses were heavy smokers, and that Brian, in particular, liked to drink a six-pack a day on summer weekends, on top of his usual three or four beers a night after work. Perhaps living right could influence their chances of pregnancy. They had some time, because they were only in their late 20s. Since trying IVF would have meant selling the boat to get the cash, Brian and Maureen felt very motivated to exhaust other options. The spouses enrolled together in a quit-smoking program at their local hospital. Brian also decided to put the money he usually spent on beer and cigarettes into a piggy bank that would be used either for IVF or for buying a new house if they had a baby. He was surprised at how much he saved over the next year. An even better surprise was the day Maureen's pregnancy test was positive. She had an uneventful pregnancy and gave birth to an 8-pound girl.

It is important to do all you can to have healthy sperm and healthy offspring. For many men with severe infertility, however, the best health habits in the world will not improve semen quality. The next chapter explains how modern techniques of assisted reproduction can help you conceive with as few as a handful of live sperm cells.

16

Using Assisted Reproductive Technology to Treat Male Infertility

Assisted reproductive technology (ART) includes infertility treatments such as intrauterine insemination (IUI), in vitro fertilization (IVF), or in vitro fertilization with intracytoplasmic sperm injection (IVF-ICSI). In these treatments, the infertility specialists use medical techniques to bypass not only sexual intercourse, but often other portions of the reproductive journey, to get the sperm to the egg.

PREPARING SPERM FOR ART

When assisted reproductive techniques are used for male infertility, the sperm cells must be specially prepared. Much of the seminal fluid can be discarded and the healthiest sperm cells isolated to use in the infertility procedure. When the sperm are placed directly into the uterus for intrauterine insemination, it is important to eliminate the *seminal plasma* (the fluid that makes up semen) because it contains chemical substances that could cause painful uterine contractions.

When the treatment of choice is IVF, the sperm are separated to concentrate the best, most motile sperm. These contenders will be layered close to the egg in a small culture dish in conventional IVF, or will become the contestants from which the embryologist will choose sperm for intracytoplasmic sperm injection (ICSI).

Although the exact details of the laboratory procedures are not crucial, couples should understand what is being done with the sperm cells and why the resulting sperm concentration and activity may be vastly different from those in the sample the husband produced and handed to the laboratory technician or embryologist.

You may hear your physician talk about "washing sperm" to prepare it for IUI or IVF. This may conjure up some strange mental images. You may be tempted to ask, "Are my sperm really that dirty? Do they need to be scrubbed clean of some bacteria or toxin? I thought I washed my hands pretty well!" Actually, washing is a misnomer. The term *sperm separation* is more accurate.

Separating the Good, the Bad, and the Ugly. A number of methods are used to separate out the best quality sperm from a single, ejaculated semen sample. The easiest, but least selective, is simply to spin the semen very rapidly in a machine called a centrifuge. The sperm cells gravitate to the bottom of a cone-shaped test tube, whereas the liquid part of the semen floats on top. The seminal fluid is sucked out of the tube, leaving a compact pellet of sperm cells. The pellet is mixed into a small amount of a special fluid—a process called resuspension. The fluid chosen contains chemicals that help sperm cells survive, but will not irritate a woman's uterus if the mixture is used for IUI.

Centrifuging the semen cannot separate live sperm cells from dead ones. In order to pick out the live sperm, more sophisticated laboratory methods are needed. When semen is first ejaculated, it coagulates, or thickens, into a semisolid, and then liquefies again. As the fluid thins out, the active sperm tend to swim to the most liquid portion. In the laboratory, a technique called the *swim-up* takes advantage of this process. The semen sample is separated into three or more portions and put into separate test tubes. The number of portions varies depending on the semen quality and amount of fluid. The technician carefully layers a few drops of a sperm-attracting, thinner fluid on top of each semen sample. This medium contains chemicals that can nourish the sperm and keep them alive. The tubes are put into an incubator set at body temperature. Over time, the sperm cells swim to the thinner medium. After an hour or two, the most active sperm cells can be siphoned off from the top layer. Unfortunately, this is not a very efficient way of separating sperm. Many of the more weakly motile sperm cells are lost in the lower layers of the test tubes. Thus the swim-up is usually reserved for situations in which a man's semen quality is excellent, but IUI is going to be used to try to bypass an infertility problem on the female side. Swim-up is also used at times on a semen sample of poorer quality when the goal is to select sperm cells for conventional IVF or IVF-ICSI.

Currently, the most efficient ways of separating out the best sperm use a special liquid with *density gradients,* or layers of varying thickness. Imagine the layers as starting out like water and ending up about the consistency of Jell-O. The sperm cells that swim the most strongly will have a better chance of reaching the most solid layer. In the laboratory, a test tube is prepared with the densest layer on the bottom and less dense layers on top. The semen sample is placed gently on the top of this mixture and the tube is spun in a centrifuge for about 20 minutes. The best quality sperm are pulled to the bottom layer, leaving most of the dead, nonmotile, or weakly motile sperm in the rest of the liquid, which can be siphoned off and discarded. The remaining pellet of highly active sperm cells is resuspended in a special solution and centrifuged again for 5 to 10 minutes. Again the upper layer is discarded and the sperm-rich bottom portion is suspended in a few drops of fluid. Now it is ready to be used for IUI or IVF. Although these laboratory techniques allow us to prepare even small or poor quality semen samples for ART, there is always some wastage of good sperm.

Cryopreserving Sperm Cells. It is sometimes helpful to have a sample of sperm cells frozen, later to be thawed and used for infertility treatment. Experts have known since the 1950s how to prepare and freeze semen. The sperm cells are placed in a protective fluid to coat their surface and prevent freezer burn. Semen samples are generally divided into small amounts for freezing and placed into plastic vials or thin, hollow containers called *straws.* Most laboratories that *cryopreserve* (freeze and store) sperm have sophisticated electronic equipment that freezes the specimens in a tank of liquid nitrogen, controlling the temperatures in a series of steps to minimize damage to the sperm cells. Laboratories also have a very strict system for labeling the samples, with double checks and logbooks to accurately identify the man who produced the sample, both at the time of freezing and when it is thawed.

Some sperm cells do not make it through the freezing and thawing process. In fact, the general rule is that "only the strong survive." Nevertheless, cryopreservation is very helpful in preserving sperm recovered surgically from the epididymis or a testicle for use in a future cycle of IVF-ICSI, which requires only a small number of live sperm. It is not helpful, however, to freeze many samples with poor semen quality, hoping to be able to collect and concentrate enough to use with IUI. As our freezing processes improve in the future, perhaps it will become possible to preserve more sperm from each sample, allowing greater freedom of choice of ART procedure.

Cryopreservation has also allowed hospital-based and commercial sperm banks to begin operating. Besides cryopreserving sperm from infertility patients, sperm banks also offer their services to men who are about to undergo cancer therapy or other types of medical treatment that might permanently damage their fertility (see chapter 14). Some men also may wish to have the added insurance of sperm in the bank before having a vasectomy. Some sperm banks also store sperm from men who agree to be sperm donors. As we discuss in the next chapter, these semen samples are sold to couples around the world who want to have a child through donor insemination.

INTRAUTERINE INSEMINATION

Intrauterine insemination is one of the more common techniques used for mild male factor infertility. This method is typically only mildly uncomfortable for a woman, and involves a brief office procedure that can be performed by a physician or a trained nurse. After preparing a semen sample as we described above, it is placed in a very small, thin tube, or *catheter.* This catheter is passed through the opening in the center of a woman's cervix. Then the washed sperm is released directly into her uterus. This procedure brings the sperm cells closer to their meeting place in the fallopian tube with the ripe egg. They do not have to swim through the mucus that coats the entrance to the cervix.

For some couples, IUI can increase the chances of fertilization. On the other hand, it has some limitations. When a man ejaculates his semen into his partner's vagina, or if a semen sample is simply placed right at the cervix, the cervical mucus acts as a filter. As the sperm cells swim through the mucus, some of the seminal fluid is naturally washed away, allowing the best quality sperm to get through. Since these sperm have a longer journey than those deposited into the uterus for IUI, they need to be in better shape (kind of like running a full marathon instead of a 10-kilometer race). The cervix also contains many crypts or nooks and crannies in which sperm gather, to be released slowly over the next day or two. These stored sperm are like a corps of reserve soldiers, replenishing the men on the front lines who are fighting to get to the egg. A supply of sperm is available for at least two days after each episode of intercourse or vaginal insemination. When IUI is done, however, the prepared sperm are only capable of fertilizing the egg for about 12 hours, making correct timing of the essence.

When a man has a moderately low sperm count and/or motility, IUI can increase the chance of pregnancy. Generally, at least 2 million motile sperm need to be recovered from the semen after preparation for IUI to have a reasonable chance of success. The forward progression of the sperm is also important. Intrauterine insemination does not work well when antisperm antibodies are present, but is a very helpful treatment if an erection problem prevents intercourse or if a man has severe, uncorrected hypospadias and cannot ejaculate into his partner's vagina. This procedure may also be used to bypass problems in the female partner; for example, if her cervical mucus does not get thin enough at ovulation to allow the sperm cells to swim through, or if the passageway through her cervix has been narrowed by scar tissue. Some recent data from our own center suggest that IUI is more successful when women are under age 36 and have not had any previous surgery in the pelvic area.

Intrauterine insemination is timed to coincide with the woman's day of ovulation or the day before she ovulates. Sometimes inseminations are performed two days in a row. The success of IUI may be increased if the woman is given oral or injectable hormones to stimulate her ovaries to ripen more than one oocyte. The combination of injectable hormone stimulation and IUI is called *superovulation*. Superovulation is a common treatment for male factor infertility when sperm counts and motility are reduced, but not so poor that IVF-ICSI is needed. It may also be used for unexplained infertility, when no clear problem has been identified in either partner.

Superovulation may be less risky than IVF for the female partner, especially if she is under age 35 and has no known infertility problem on her side. Compared to an IVF cycle, doses of hormones are lower for superovulation, reducing the risk of overstimulating the ovaries, which can cause a serious medical crisis, as we describe below (see page 146). On the other hand, it is harder to control the risks of multiple births with superovulation than it is with IVF. If ultrasounds show that too many follicles are developing around the time of ovulation, the insemination can be canceled. Either the couple can try a new cycle with lower doses of hormones for the woman, or the oocytes can be harvested and fertilized in the laboratory, converting the IUI cycle to IVF, with the opportunity to transfer only two or three embryos.

If three cycles of superovulation fail to result in a pregnancy when a couple has male factor or combination factor infertility, many infertility specialists would advocate going on to try in vitro fertilization. Very few pregnancies occur in couples with male factor infertility after six unsuccessful superovulation cycles.

IN VITRO FERTILIZATION

In vitro fertilization can be used to treat a variety of types of infertility, including problems on the female side, the male side, or unexplained infertility. Fertilization of the egg takes place in the laboratory. To prepare a woman's ovaries for IVF, she is often given drugs that interrupt her menstrual cycle, creating a temporary menopause for a couple of weeks. Then she begins a series of daily hormone shots that stimulate her ovaries to ripen multiple eggs. The progress of the cycle is monitored by testing her blood for the levels of the hormone estrogen, and by scanning her pelvis with an ultrasound machine to measure the number and size of ovarian follicles (remember that a follicle is a nest of cells and fluid that contains the ripening egg) that are developing.

When the growing size of the follicles signals that ovulation is near, the woman is given a shot of human chorionic gonadotropin (HCG), a hormone that helps the oocytes finish maturing. The next day, she undergoes an outpatient surgical procedure called *transvaginal ultrasound-guided follicle aspiration*. She usually will be put under a light anesthesia, or at least given sedatives and pain medication to make the procedure more comfortable. The reproductive endocrinologist uses an ultrasound image of the patient's ovaries to aim a thin needle into each follicle. The fluid inside the follicle and the oocyte are sucked out with a syringe and brought immediately to the embryology laboratory. The eggs are processed and each is placed in a sterile dish with a nutrient solution. Sperm cells are added to the eggs after the material surrounding the egg "shells" has been removed. Typically 50,000 to 100,000 sperm cells are added to a dish if a man has good semen quality, and up to 1 million with each egg if semen quality is poor.

If an egg fertilizes, the resulting embryo is allowed to continue to grow and divide for two or three days. The couple and their medical team decide how many embryos should be transferred back into the woman's uterus. Transferring embryos is a simple office procedure. The embryos are still microscopic in size. They are placed in a catheter, which is passed through the cervix so that the embryos can be flushed out into the woman's uterine cavity. The team checks the catheter afterwards to make sure all the embryos were placed inside the uterus.

Traditionally, embryos have been transferred after two or three days of growth in the laboratory. Recently, IVF programs have begun to try to culture embryos for five to seven days until they reach a stage in which they are called blastocysts. At this time the embryo begins to form a tiny, hollow ball of cells. When blastocysts are transferred back into the uterus, the rate of implantation and pregnancy is typically higher than when earlier stage embryos are used. The downside is that some embryos may die in the laboratory instead of continuing to become blastocysts. Researchers believe that most of these embryos are of poor quality and would not have been able to implant and create a pregnancy if they had been placed into the uterus at an earlier stage.

The biggest advantage of using blastocysts is that fewer embryos can be transferred, but with as good or better pregnancy rates and a much reduced risk of triplet or higher order multiple pregnancies. Culturing embryos to blastocyst stage requires a very skilled IVF laboratory, however, and not all programs offer this option. Blastocysts also may not survive cryopreservation as well as very early embryos do. Many IVF programs prefer to freeze several embryos very early in the culturing process, allowing the remainder to grow to the blastocyst stage. Obviously these choices work best when a number of fertilized eggs are available.

INTRACYTOPLASMIC
SPERM INJECTION

Men who are infertile typically have low sperm counts and motility, resulting in poor rates of fertilization even when conventional IVF is performed. In 1992, the technique of intracytoplasmic sperm injection was introduced, revolutionizing the success rates of IVF with male factor infertility. In ICSI, the embryologist uses a special robotic microscope to actually catch a sperm cell. Careful preparation of sperm is especially important when using ICSI. Sperm samples are washed and the most motile sperm are isolated. The sperm cell is injected into the egg using a hollow glass needle. Performing ICSI is a learned skill, and you want an embryologist who has performed at least 100 procedures. As the embryologist's skill improves, she or he can typically achieve at least 60 percent rates of fertilization. These rates are similar to those achieved when a man has good semen quality, or perhaps a little better.

Because the women in couples who use IVF-ICSI often have normal fertility and are younger than many other women who have IVF, pregnancy rates have been better than those using conventional IVF for a range of infertility problems. For example, in the year 1995, data from the report of the Society for Assisted Reproductive Technology show that for cycles using ICSI in couples with male factor infertility, 27.2 percent of cycles in which eggs were retrieved ended with the live birth of a baby. This compares to 21.5 percent of IVF cycles without ICSI when a male factor was the primary diagnosis. A number of the larger and more successful IVF programs around the country report even better live birth rates than these when ICSI is used and the woman is under age 35 with no known female infertility.

These young, fertile women are also at higher risk for *ovarian hyperstimulation,* however. When this complication of IVF occurs, the level of estrogen in a woman's bloodstream shoots up and her ovaries swell. Mild hyperstimulation can often be controlled by stopping hormone shots for several days during the IVF cycle. If hyperstimulation persists, the eggs can still be harvested when mature and fertilized in the lab, but any embryos that result are frozen rather than being transferred. The embryos can be thawed and replaced in a future month, when hormone levels have normalized.

Beginning a pregnancy in a state of ovarian hyperstimulation can quickly escalate the problem. If hyperstimulation is severe, fluid builds up in a woman's pelvis and lungs, making her very ill. Hospitalization is required to manage this crisis, and death can even result, although this happens rarely. Not only are younger and more fertile women more at risk for hyperstimulation, but also women who are petite and thin, making it more difficult to regulate their hormone dose properly.

GETTING THE SPERM FOR IVF-ICSI
FROM THE EPIDIDYMIS OR A TESTICLE

Most men with fertility problems have at least some live sperm cells in their semen. As long as even a few live sperm cells are available in a semen sample, they can be used for ICSI. Some men will not have any sperm cells in their semen, however. Some of these men have dry ejaculations, in which no fluid spurts out at climax. In chapter 13 we discussed using medication, vibrator stimulation, or electroejaculation to enable these men to ejaculate semen. Most of the semen samples obtained in these ways contain enough sperm for ICSI. The procedure can also be performed using sperm retrieved from a man's urine, as chapter 13 describes.

Some men ejaculate seminal fluid at the moment of orgasm, but it contains no live sperm cells. Some of these men have a blockage of the sperm pathways in the epididymis, or were born without the vas deferens. Some have had vasectomies or failed attempts to reverse a vasectomy. A few may have had the prostate and the seminal vesicles removed as part of a cancer operation. In these situations, where the testicles make normal amounts of sperm cells, spermatozoa can be retrieved in a variety of ways, depending on the experience of the surgeon and the patient's preference. *Microsurgical epididymal sperm aspiration* (MESA) is a common method used to obtain sperm when a man has blocked sperm pathways and either is not a good candidate for reconstructive surgery or chooses MESA instead. The surgeon exposes the epididymis through an incision made in the scrotum. Viewing the epididymis at high magnification through an operating microscope, the surgeon opens a single loop of the epididymal tubule. Sperm cells are aspirated (sucked out) through this opening and sent to the embryologist. The advantage of MESA is that extra sperm are usually available for freezing, in case IVF-ICSI needs to be repeated in the future.

Some physicians prefer to aspirate the sperm by placing a needle into the epididymis or the testis through the skin, using a local anesthetic to numb the area. This procedure has the advantage that it can be done in a doctor's office, but the disadvantage is that it does not usually yield a large enough number of sperm cells to freeze extra samples. As we describe in chapter 5, an open biopsy of the testicle can also be used to obtain sperm for IVF-ICSI. Small bits of tissue from the biopsy can be frozen, and thawed at another time to allow the embryologist to find live sperm cells. Successful freezing of tissue from the testicle requires an experienced laboratory, however.

The situation becomes more complex if a man's testicles produce very few sperm cells—for example, in some genetic infertility syndromes. Sometimes no sperm cell production is taking place. In other cases, tiny scattered islands of sperm production exist, even though no sperm is found in the semen. If several samples of testicular tissue are taken out during a testicular biopsy, the laboratory may be able to find a few live, mature sperm cells to use in ICSI. This procedure is known as TESE, for *testicular sperm extraction*. Tissue from the biopsy is minced up and put in a solution. It is a tedious process to examine this solution to find sperm. Sometimes it takes hours to find any. If no mature sperm cells are found, immature round spermatids have sometimes been used for ICSI. Although this is controversial, no unusual rate of birth defects has resulted in the few babies born thus far.

When a testicular biopsy done for the sake of diagnosis showed some sperm cell production in the past, it is usually worthwhile to try TESE on the day of the woman's egg retrieval. Some couples may wish to have semen from a donor available as a backup, however, in case the husband's tissue fails to yield any sperm. Couples may feel that they do not want to waste the chance to have a baby, especially if they had planned to use donor insemination if IVF failed. Other couples would just not be comfortable having a child through donor insemination and choose to end IVF at that point, or to freeze the woman's eggs for a future procedure, even though egg freezing is experimental. Some couples who plan to try donor insemination using IUI in the event of an IVF failure prefer to skip donor backup for IVF. They do not think it is worth taking the risk of multiple pregnancies from an IVF embryo transfer.

OTHER ART METHODS

You may be offered other variations of ART. Some programs use *gamete intrafallopian transfer,* or GIFT. In this procedure, the woman undergoes ovarian stimulation and has her ripe oocytes harvested. The eggs and sperm are then deposited into her fallopian tubes. The hope for GIFT was that fertilization would take place in the tubes, and because this would be more "natural," pregnancy rates would be higher. Unfortunately, a laparoscopy is needed to perform GIFT, making it more expensive and harder on the woman. A variation of GIFT is *zygote intrafallopian transfer,* or ZIFT, in which an embryo created in the laboratory is inserted into the fallopian tube rather than through the cervix and into the uterus. The success rates for GIFT or ZIFT have not proved superior enough to justify the additional surgery, and these treatments have lost popularity. Some Catholic couples choose GIFT, however, because it is considered acceptable by some religious scholars whereas IVF is not condoned by the church (see page 151).

Another variation of ART is the use of *assisted hatching* with IVF. After embryos form, the embryologist creates a tiny opening in the outer layer of cells. Assisted hatching is believed to help the embryo to implant in the uterine lining, particularly when the woman in the couple is in her late 30s or early 40s. Assisted hatching remains controversial, however, and its effectiveness is unproven.

FINDING AN ART PROGRAM
YOU CAN TRUST

The media suggest that infertility patients should take the attitude *"caveat emptor,"* or "buyer beware," when dealing with ART clinics. It is true that regulations of the infertility health industry are somewhat loose, just as they are in general with medicine in the United States compared to European countries. Indeed, there have been cases of infertility clinics misrepresenting their success rates, mixing up people's gametes and embryos, deliberately giving away eggs to a second couple without permission, or acting in other unscrupulous ways. Since a majority of people pay for some or all of their infertility treatment out of their pocket, there is always the possibility of undeserved profits for the clinics and tragic emotional and financial losses for vulnerable men and women who long for a baby. While we do believe that the majority of infertility clinics in the United States treat couples in an ethical manner, it is very wise to be cautious. Here are some ways to check out a clinic.

Ask if a program meets the American Society for Reproductive Medicine (ASRM) guidelines and has a laboratory accredited by the College of American Pathologists and the ASRM. Find out whether the reproductive endocrinologists in the program are board certified in their specialty. You can also find out specific success rates for the program if it reports its yearly statistics to the Society for Assisted Reproductive Technology (SART). Although participation in SART is voluntary, the great majority of the most successful and established infertility clinics in the United States do so. You can order SART reports through Resolve or ASRM, or view them on the web site of the Centers for Disease Control (CDC) (see "Resources" for more information). The reports are organized by state and actually give you specific data on pregnancy rates for each clinic, including numbers and types of ART cycles performed, cycles canceled, average number of embryos transferred, pregnancy rates per cycle, and pregnancy rates per embryo transfer. Reports give separate listings by the woman's age or whether a male factor was involved. Recently, ICSI data is reported separately from that of conventional IVF.

You want to find a clinic that is experienced, even more so if ICSI is involved. Look at the length of time the clinic has been in operation, and the number of IVF cycles of different types completed in the past year. Even using SART reports, comparing pregnancy rates between programs is tricky, since some clinics may have a mix of couples who are younger, with causes of infertility, such as tubal disease, that yield the highest IVF success rates. Some clinics transfer more than three embryos per cycle, perhaps increasing their pregnancy rates slightly, but also yielding higher rates of multiple pregnancies with all the risks that go with them. Some clinics have very good pregnancy rates with fresh embryos, but poor rates with frozen and thawed embryos. That can be a real handicap if your cycle goes well, but a pregnancy does not result with the fresh transfer.

The SART report is usually about three years behind the current date. If you are interested in a particular clinic, call them and ask for their most recent statistics, to make sure they still are as successful as in the past. A change of staff or a problem with the embryology laboratory can quickly sink a good program.

Ask, too, about the costs of the program, including the drugs that are part of the cycle. If you have to pay in advance, will the whole amount be due? Are you responsible for the cost of a full cycle even if it is canceled before egg recovery or if no embryos are available for transfer? How helpful is the clinic in submitting bills to your insurance company, including billing some items separately, such as laboratory tests or ultrasounds, that may be covered even if your insurance excludes IVF itself?

RELIGIOUS ISSUES AND ART

The major world religions have commented on the morality and acceptability of using technology to help conception. As you might expect, different religions have very disparate ideas about ART. See table on next page.

THE HEALTH OF CHILDREN BORN FROM ART

Although working with sperm cells and oocytes in the laboratory seems like the kind of thing that might promote birth defects, there is little evidence that children born from ART have increased health problems. The

Religion	Opinions about ART	Reason for the Opinion
Catholic Church	IUI is not allowed. IVF is not allowed. Embryo cryo-preservation is not allowed. GIFT is debatable, if semen is collected surgical-ly or via a collection condom during sex-ual intercourse.	Conception should take place during an act of marital inter-course, and this moral principle is violated if concep-tion takes place in the laboratory. The embryo is consid-ered a new life from the moment of fer-tilization and should be treated with all the respect due a liv-ing human being.
Protestant Churches	Most Protestant Churches do not object to IUI or IVF. Churches that view the embryo as a new life may reject cryo-preservation or destruction of embryos.	Protestant denomi-nations that do not condone ART or embryo storage tend to use similar rea-sons as those on which Catholic opin-ion is based.
Judaism	IUI is permitted, but Orthodox Jews need to wait for several years of marriage to show that other means will not work, or have a medically sound rationale. Insemination should only be done during the same parts of the wife's cycle when intercourse would be permitted. It is bet-ter to obtain semen	

continued

Table *Continued*

Religion	Opinions about ART	Reason for the Opinion
Judaism *continued*	during intercourse rather than through masturbation. Orthodox rabbis differ on IVF, but most permit it. A few believe that the children born are no longer the legal offspring of the parents, however. Conservative and reform rabbis condone ART.	
Islam	IUI and IVF are permitted if the sperm and oocytes come from members of a married couple. Cryopreservation of embryos is allowed, but embryos have to be transferred to the same wife during a valid marriage.	It is crucial to assure that the child is the genetic offspring of both mother and father in the married couple.

procedures used today do not seem to damage chromosomes directly. Because ART results in more multiple pregnancies, complications related to having twins, triplets, or even higher-order births must be considered, including low birth weights for the infants, premature labor and birth, stillbirth, and an increased rate of cerebral palsy or learning problems seen when very low-birth-weight babies survive to grow up. Singleton babies born from IUI or IVF are at little or no greater health risk than babies conceived through sexual intercourse. The possibility that using IVF-ICSI could transmit genetic problems was discussed in detail in chapter 7. So far, the studies of children born from this technology have been, by and large, reassuring.

RIDING THE EMOTIONAL
ROLLER COASTER OF ART

When infertility treatment involves ART, each cycle can become an emotional roller coaster. At the start, you cannot help feeling a spark of hope that this treatment will be the one that gives you a baby. Since ART always involves some hassles and discomforts, not to mention financial expense, you need some optimism to carry you through the procedures. During the cycle, your mood may be affected by the feedback you get. How many follicles are developing? How are the estrogen levels? Each piece of news can raise your expectations or bring on a black funk. At the end of a cycle, you react to the outcome: depression if no pregnancy results and joy if there is a positive test. Even when a pregnancy occurs, however, there is the high risk of early miscarriage. An ultrasound showing a fetal heartbeat is reassuring, but for many couples, the anxiety does not stop until they take the baby home from the hospital (and maybe not even then).

HOW STRESSFUL IS ART?

Most couples who begin ART treatments have already experienced a complex evaluation for infertility. Many have tried for months or years to conceive through intercourse, with increasing disappointment each cycle. A number of research studies show that people with infertility are not especially likely to have a true case of depression or panic disorder, but do commonly report specific distress about getting pregnant.

How stressful is ART? Compared to a cycle of trying to conceive naturally, women undergoing IVF reported feeling more optimistic and having more physical discomfort, but the amount of extra stress they experienced was not very striking. In fact, most couples cope reasonably well with the stress of ART. Those who begin infertility treatment with other life issues that have made them unusually depressed or anxious, or with significant tension in their marriage, often can use some extra counseling during a treatment cycle. You yourself are probably the best judge of your own stress level, but sometimes others around you, including your spouse, may point out that you are unusually irritable or withdrawn. Then it may be helpful to ask your infertility specialist to refer you to a mental health professional who is familiar with infertility treatment and its emotional side effects.

Another confusing issue is the impact of the hormones that are given to women during many ART cycles, including drugs that cause temporary menopause and oral and injectable drugs that stimulate ovulation. Many women experience depression or irritability as medication side effects, although it is difficult to predict how a hormone medication will impact on any individual. Some women notice little change in their moods while on the medications. Others feel "out of control," and may even worry that their distress will decrease their chances of pregnancy.

DOES STRESS INTERFERE
WITH ART PREGNANCY?

Many couples worry that feeling stressed out during infertility treatment will in itself prevent pregnancy from taking place. A number of self-help books reinforce this idea, and suggest that having psychotherapy, or at least using stress management techniques such as relaxation routines or meditation, will improve your chances of getting pregnant. Psychologists have theorized that severe depression or anxiety may interfere with ovulation or with implantation of the embryo. Chemicals in the brain that affect a woman's moods may also be able to influence the hormones controlling her menstrual cycle. Yet there is actually very little scientific evidence that a woman's state of mind interferes with pregnancy, especially when her hormones are being controlled by infertility treatment.

One of the most careful studies of emotions and pregnancy during IVF asked women to keep daily diaries of their moods and symptoms. Women who did not get pregnant indeed reported more negative moods. When the researchers looked back, however, they discovered that the women's moods in the failed IVF group only differed from those of the IVF success group on the days that they received feedback about how the cycle was going. Women in the failed IVF group were having medical problems with their cycles, and reacted with depression and anxiety to the bad news. Not surprisingly, the strong predictors of pregnancy were the medical factors in IVF. The emotional differences between the two groups probably resulted from awareness of the medical glitches, and were not causes in themselves of IVF failure.

Another way to look at stress and pregnancy is to think of the many women who become pregnant during wartime or famine. If stress played a very large role in pregnancy, one would not expect to see pregnant women in those situations. In fact, about 5 percent of rapes of young women end in unwanted pregnancy, and it is difficult to imagine a more stressful way of conceiving than that!

On the other hand, research does suggest that experiencing very stressful life events during early pregnancy may contribute to miscarriage or to the mother's having health problems during the pregnancy. Still, rates of miscarriage after ART are similar to those expected in any attempt to conceive. Up to a third of all very early pregnancies end in miscarriage. When a couple has not been trying systematically to conceive, they often are never aware of these miscarriages. The woman may simply notice that her menstrual period came a little bit late. Pregnancy tests after an ART cycle are typically performed as early as possible, however, so that all *chemical pregnancies* (the first sign, marked by a rise in the hormone beta HCG, that the embryo has implanted into the uterine lining) are identified.

We usually suggest that when couples get a positive pregnancy test after an ART cycle, they wait several weeks to share the results with all but their closest family members or friends. If an early miscarriage does occur, it just adds to your heartbreak to have to inform all of the people who were so glad to share your joy about the pregnancy. By around week six or seven, when a fetal heartbeat can be seen on ultrasound, the greatest danger of miscarriage is over, and you may feel ready to let more people in on your news.

COPING WITH STRESS
DURING AN ART CYCLE

It is just common sense to try to reduce your stress during an ART cycle. Coming back and forth to the infertility clinic for blood tests or ultrasounds, or having daily hormone injections, is hassle enough. If you can reduce your working hours, avoid heavy physical labor, or distance yourself from conflict-laden relationships during those weeks, your life will be easier. Stress management techniques such as practicing relaxation skills at least once a day can also help you cope with the stress of ART. Some relaxation routines ask you to focus on your breathing as you mentally repeat a cue word, such as "calm" or "relax." Others guide you in imagining a relaxing scene, such as picturing yourself lying on the soft sand of a tropical beach. Another very effective technique is called progressive muscle relaxation, and involves tensing and relaxing the different groups of muscles in your body. You can learn relaxation techniques by purchasing commercially available audiotapes or videotapes, or by attending a group or individual session with a trained mental health professional.

Some couples or individual partners benefit from being part of a support group during an ART cycle. Some groups provide information or discussion in an educational format. Others are more like therapy groups and encourage members to share their emotional experiences with each other. Some infertility clinics provide special groups for ART couples. Many cities have a local chapter of Resolve (see "Resources") that organizes groups.

Providing mutual understanding and tolerance is very important for partners in a couple going through an ART cycle. If the woman flies off the handle over some small issue that would not normally bother her, both of you need to remember that the hormones she is taking may be affecting her patience. You can help each other in making sure you take medications on time, learn how to give injections, interpret your ovulation kit correctly, keep your doctor appointments, and generally follow all the complicated instructions you have been given. In an IVF cycle, perhaps the most emotionally trying time is the two weeks of waiting for a pregnancy test once embryos have been transferred to the woman's uterus. This is often a good time to plan some enjoyable activities to take your mind off of IVF—for example, going to funny movies, getting away for the weekend, or doing some other leisure activity you especially enjoy.

COPING WITH ART FAILURE

Even in a very good infertility program, a couple typically faces a higher chance of failure with any cycle of ART than of going home with a baby. Several studies have shown that despite being informed of these statistics, couples typically believe that they will be among the lucky minority who achieve pregnancy. Perhaps couples need that kind of optimism to gamble their energy, time, and money on an ART cycle.

Studies of the impact of ART failure have largely been based on couples trying IVF. Since IVF is usually close to the end of the line, as far as infertility treatments go, a failure may be especially distressing. Repeated failures of intrauterine insemination, with or without ovary-stimulating drugs, can also be very wearing, however. The group most vulnerable to depression seems to be childless women. Symptoms not uncommon after failed IVF include trouble sleeping or eating, nightmares, panic attacks, or even thoughts of suicide. If such problems persist more than a couple of days, it is important to seek help from a physician or counselor.

COPING WITH THE RISK
OF MULTIPLE BIRTHS

Whenever ART involves giving a woman drugs to stimulate her ovulation, there is an increased risk of multiple births. In the industrialized nations, rates of multiple pregnancy have increased dramatically since the 1970s. Births of triplets and higher have doubled. An estimate within the United States is that 38 percent of triplet and higher births occur because of ART, whereas 30 percent are due to childbearing by older women who are more likely to have multiple pregnancies. Risks to the health of mothers and infants because of multiple pregnancies are the most important negative outcomes of ART.

Couples using ART typically feel very positive about the idea of having twins. They often say it would be "two for the price of one" or would mean they would be finished with their family and would not have to repeat infertility treatment. Studies suggest that at least half of ART couples would even welcome triplets.

Unfortunately, the medical outcome of multiple pregnancies is not as positive as couples might hope. Even with twins, health problems during pregnancy such as preeclampsia (high blood pressure), gestational diabetes, premature birth, and low-birth-weight babies are more common. With triplets, outcomes are poor enough that some physcians may offer selective reduction of the pregnancy to twins, which may lead to fewer premature deliveries, bigger babies, and fewer health problems for the mothers.

Selective reduction is a form of abortion involving the injection of a fatal dose of a chemical into one or more fetuses, early in a multiple pregnancy. Usually triplet or higher order pregnancies are reduced to twin pregnancies. There is some risk of miscarrying the remaining fetuses, but most women are able to continue the pregnancy. Psychological studies of women who chose selective reduction find that they initially feel a good deal of guilt and grief. After a brief time, however, 93 percent in one study felt they would make the same decision again, and long-term psychological distress is rare.

The best way to avoid agonizing choices about selective reduction is to prevent multiple pregnancies from ART. Intrauterine insemination cycles should be canceled if too many follicles are developing, or the eggs can be harvested and fertilized in the laboratory, changing over to IVF. With IVF-ICSI, couples often include a wife of normal fertility and under age 35. In this situation, couples should consider transferring only two embryos rather than three, to minimize the risk of triplets. Extra embryos can be frozen for transfer in a future cycle. As success rates for IVF continue to increase, and especially with new technology that allows embryos to grow in the lab to the more advanced blastocyst stage before being transferred, limiting transfers to two embryos will be increasingly common.

MAKING CHOICES
ABOUT FREEZING EMBRYOS

Typically, infertility specialists hope that one cycle of IVF will result in enough embryos so that a fresh embryo transfer can take place, and extras can be frozen (cryopreserved) for transfer at a later date, either if no pregnancy results on the fresh cycle, or if the couple wants to have another child in the future. Some couples feel comfortable creating embryos with IVF, but have religious or ethical concerns about freezing embryos, or about potentially leaving some frozen embryos unused. Programs typically give couples the option of having unused frozen embryos destroyed, or donating them to another couple with infertility who would essentially adopt the genetically unrelated embryo and attempt to carry it to term.

At least in the United States, couples more commonly destroy unused embryos and are reluctant to donate them, feeling uncomfortable with the idea of having a genetically related child alive somewhere, but unknown to them. One exception is that couples who create embryos with donated eggs from an anonymous volunteer donor are much more likely to donate any leftover embryos to another couple.

Some couples with male factor infertility choose to avoid the issue by not freezing embryos. Their most typical option is to try *natural cycle IVF,* in which the woman's ovulation is monitored, but she is given either no stimulating hormones, or a very small dose. The hope is to harvest one or a very few ripe eggs, fertilize them using ICSI, and then replace only one or two embryos. The drawback is that natural cycle IVF is almost as expensive as conventional IVF. The main cost you avoid is that of the hormone medications. Pregnancy rates, however, are quite low, typically less than 10 percent per cycle. Another option is to use limited hormone stimulation, aiming at producing at least two or three embryos to use on a fresh cycle.

If you are having a difficult time making choices about freezing embryos, you may want to talk to a religious counselor you can trust, or to a bioethicist—an expert in the ethical choices involved in medical practice. Your infertility program may be able to suggest some resource people in your community who have been of help to other couples experiencing this dilemma.

Now we move from the highest of high-tech to a treatment for infertility that has been in use for most of the past century—donor insemination. It is also a move from the most expensive end of the spectrum to the most economical way to have a baby when a man has infertility problems.

17

Having a Child through Donor Insemination

Of all the treatments available for male infertility, using sperm from a donor to conceive a child is the most controversial. The positive aspects of donor insemination are very clear. It is probably the least expensive way to conceive a baby, other than through natural intercourse. If there is no fertility problem on the female side, most couples will achieve a pregnancy within four to six cycles, using a simple, painless procedure performed in the doctor's office. The wife has the chance to experience pregnancy, ensure that she has excellent prenatal care, and contribute her genes to a child. When couples use a sperm donor from a reputable sperm bank, they know the donor's family background was screened for genetic diseases, and that the donor was healthy himself. Most donors are also reasonably attractive and intelligent young men. The donor can be matched to the husband on physical traits and ethnicity. If the husband carries a genetic problem that could affect the health of his offspring, using a donor avoids this risk. Follow-up studies of families that have had a child through donor insemination suggest that the children are healthy and well-adjusted, and that the parents love and value them tremendously.

Donor insemination's negative aspects are more emotional, and sometimes ethical or spiritual. Choosing this option means that a couple gives up their dream of creating a mutual, genetic child as the living symbol and fulfillment of their love for each other. The father may not feel quite the same pride or connection as he would have with his own biological child. It is possible that a child created via donor insemination will be more different from the father than a mutual genetic child would have been, for example, in specific talents, appearance, or basic personality style. The mother, too, often feels disappointment at being unable to carry the child of the man she loves. Conceiving a child in the doctor's office using sperm cells from a stranger can be an alienating process, depending on how the husband and wife view it. In addition, the Catholic Church, Islam, and most rabbis in Orthodox Judaism reject donor insemination as an option to treat infertility, as we discuss later in this chapter.

EMOTIONAL REACTIONS TO DONOR INSEMINATION

Many couples reject donor insemination as an option right off the bat. Often it is the man who is afraid he could never love a baby that was not his genetic child. Women also commonly feel they only want to carry the child of the man they love. Sometimes one or both partners sees adoption as a fairer choice, since neither parent then has a genetic relationship to the child. Donor insemination remains a very viable way to have a child, however, for couples with male infertility who can accept the idea.

THE PROCESS OF MAKING A CHOICE

Donor insemination is not something to choose on impulse. When couples fall in love and marry, the great majority expect to become parents through uncomplicated sexual intercourse. They imagine how the mother's and father's physical traits, personality strengths and flaws, and talents may combine to create a unique and precious child. Unless a couple knows about male infertility before the partners make a commitment to each other, donor insemination is not even on their radar screen as a way to build a family.

Most mental health professionals who work with infertile couples recommend that a husband and wife take their time in deciding on donor insemination. Part of that process is coming to terms with the news of severe male infertility and grieving for the mutual genetic child that will never be. Another aspect is making a decision between donor insemination and alternatives such as trying IVF-ICSI (in vitro fertilization with intracytoplasmic injection), remaining childless, or adopting.

Part of the decision process is sharing your hopes and fears about donor insemination with each other. Another part should be to meet with a mental health counselor to discuss the emotional aspects of donor insemination. You also need to be sure you can be comfortable with the religious or spiritual issues involved.

DONOR INSEMINATION IN THE UNITED STATES: PAST AND PRESENT

Donor insemination was in use in the United States as a treatment for infertility as early as the 1880s, but was not discussed in the medical literature until the 1950s. Most early donor inseminations were performed with freshly ejaculated sperm by gynecologists who used medical students or residents (or occasionally themselves) as anonymous sperm donors. Couples were told little or nothing about the donor, and were routinely counseled never to tell their child or anyone else about this mode of conception. There was no federal or state regulation of donor insemination.

By 1974, however, the American Bar Association published a model law assuring that when husband and wife in a married couple gave written consent to donor insemination, any resulting child would be considered the legal offspring of the husband, and not of the donor. Laws based on this model have been adopted by about half of American states.

When sperm freezing techniques were perfected in the 1970s, commercial sperm banks were opened. A sperm donor could give enough semen samples to establish a number of pregnancies, and these vials of semen could be stored indefinitely. Sperm banks recruit their donors not only from medical schools, but from college campuses, graduate school programs, and now the Internet. Donors are paid to undergo medical tests and provide semen samples, typically involving 9 to 12 months of weekly contacts. Their earnings can total several thousand dollars. Some private physicians still continue to recruit their own local donors, however, and they are not always as carefully screened for health and family medical history as those recruited by large sperm banks. The last government survey of sperm donation in the United States was done in 1987. At that time, 33,000 children a year were born through donor insemination.

In the mid 1980s, however, the practice of donor insemination was changed forever by the discovery of the human immunodeficiency virus (HIV) that causes AIDS. A few cases of AIDS have apparently been transmitted through the semen of a donor, although almost all of these occurred before the availability and use of HIV testing. The American Society for Reproductive Medicine (then called the American Fertility Society) issued guidelines in 1988 to ensure that semen from donors was not contaminated with HIV, or with other less lethal but still very serious sexually transmitted viruses or bacteria. Potential donors were not only to be interviewed carefully about their family medical history and their lifestyles, including use of street drugs and having unprotected sexual contacts, but were to be tested for HIV as well as a variety of other sexually transmitted diseases (STDs) as part of their screening. Then their donated semen would be frozen, and six months after the last sample was donated, the donor had to return and be retested before his semen could be released for use by couples.

Most donor semen is used in intrauterine insemination. The semen is prepared and concentrated as we discussed in the previous chapter, and then placed directly into a woman's uterus in a simple office procedure. In our clinic, a cycle of donor insemination, including the costs of purchasing the sample from a sperm bank, preparing it, and doing the insemination, costs a little over $400. Because semen quality decreases somewhat when a sample is frozen and thawed, the chance of a pregnancy on any one cycle in a woman of normal fertility is about 10 percent to 15 percent. The average woman needs four to six cycles of insemination to become pregnant. If a woman has problems with her fertility, donor semen is sometimes used with superovulation or in vitro fertilzation (IVF) procedures (see chapter 16).

Several trends have affected donor insemination in recent years. The American Society for Reproductive Medicine (ASRM) has changed its guidelines to allow directed sperm donation; that is, a couple's using a family member or friend as donor. Known sperm donors are recommended to undergo the same medical screening, however, including STD testing and quarantine of semen, as anonymous donors.

Mental health professionals have also advocated being more open with children about their origins. As donor insemination has become a topic discussed on television and in a number of books, the stigma and secrecy associated with this option have waned. Couples have begun asking for more information about the donors. Some simply want assurance that the donor's health has been fully checked out. Others want information to pass on to their children who may be curious about their biological heritage. Sperm banks have begun providing full family medical histories, and sometimes even personal statements from the donor about his hobbies, talents, and motivation to donate sperm. A very few sperm banks have a small number of donors who are willing to be identified to their adult offspring (see "Resources").

FINDING A HIGH-QUALITY SPERM BANK

As a consumer, it is very important to realize that many guidelines and standards for sperm banks are voluntary. Sperm banks do not have to follow the guidelines of the American Society for Reproductive Medicine, or be inspected and accredited by the American Association of Tissue Banks (AATB) in order to operate. They only have to meet any state or federal laws relevant to their practice. Your best protection, if you choose to use donor semen, is to work with a sperm bank that is fully accredited by the AATB. Because AATB accreditation is very rigorous and involves significant expense, a number of sperm banks have not gone through the process, but claim to follow the AATB guidelines. Other important criteria for a sperm bank include following ASRM guidelines, being licensed by its state, having a laboratory that meets CLIA (Clinical Laboratory Improvement Amendments of 1988) standards, having a medical geneticist on staff, and providing some additional services such as genetic testing of donors.

Under the latest guidelines from the AATB and the ASRM, donors are tested and retested after a minimum semen quarantine of six months for HIV-1, HIV-2, hepatitis B and C, a virus called HTLV-1 that may cause leukemia in humans, a virus called CMV (cytomegalovirus) that can cause pneumonia or encephalitis, syphilis, gonorrhea, and chlamydia. Donors must be under age 39 unless their physician permits them to participate at an older age. The sperm bank must have someone perform a physical examination and take complete medical, social, sexual, family, and genetic histories for each donor candidate. Standards for the quality of semen (sperm count, motility, etc.) that is to be stored from a donor have also been set. The AATB also recommends, but does not mandate, that in addition to completing a three-generation genetic history questionnaire, donors have genetic testing to rule out any diseases common in their ethnic group, such as cystic fibrosis gene abnormalities in Caucasians, sickle cell in African Americans, Tay-Sachs testing for Jewish donors, or thalassemia testing for donors of Mediterranean descent.

Reputable sperm banks limit the number of pregnancies produced from any one donor. A typical limit is ten offspring, although this total is sometimes stretched when a family wishes to use the same donor to conceive more than one child. The reason to limit offspring is to reduce the risk that a child born through donor insemination could one day grow up and unwittingly marry his or her half sibling. Although the chance of such an event is tiny, couples often worry about it. It may be more of a concern if couples belong to a small ethnic group and use a donor from their hometown.

Another sign of a high-quality sperm bank is that it keeps in touch with its donors and asks them to report any health problems that develop in themselves or other family members that could signal an unsuspected genetic risk to their donor offspring. Sperm banks should also keep records of any birth defects or health problems in children born from their donors, so any possible measures can be taken to prevent another such event.

FINDING SPERM DONORS
ON THE INTERNET

Recently, several sites on the Internet have begun offering whole stables of semen donors. Several of the larger sperm banks offer a catalog of their available donors that can be accessed over the Internet. Other sites act as brokers, allowing couples to advertise for specific donor characteristics, offering donors who (for an additional fee) are willing to take IQ or personality tests, or even offering fresh donors whose semen has not been frozen and quarantined (although this violates guidelines for donor insemination). Not only American couples, but couples from all over the world are using these resources to order semen because of the looser regulations in the United States compared to many European and Middle Eastern countries. It may be convenient to use the Internet to compare resources available through large, certified sperm banks. They often have the biggest pools of donors from less common ethnic backgrounds, and it is reassuring to couples to use a donor who is not from their local community to avoid even the remote possibility that their child would unwittingly someday marry a relative.

Your infertility clinic or physician may already have a contractual relationship with a particular sperm bank, however, limiting your options unless you want to find someone else to perform the inseminations. In such contracts, the sperm bank assumes legal liability in case something goes wrong—for example, if a child is born with a genetic disorder that should have been apparent from the family history or genetic testing. In fact, the rate of birth defects among children born from donor insemination is slightly less than that in the general population, probably because the donors are carefully screened.

Internet sites that charge a fee to unite you with the perfect donor can be legitimate, but be very aware of the pitfalls. The fees they charge may be quite a bit higher than those of most sperm banks. If they offer counseling for you and the donor, make sure the mental health professional is fully credentialed and trained, including being licensed appropriately in the state where the clinic is located. Some nurses or counselors may not be fully qualified. Although theoretically pregnancy rates are higher with fresh semen compared to frozen semen, your safety cannot be guaranteed. The donor can be tested for HIV using a procedure that finds the viral DNA with a technology called polymerase chain reaction (PCR), which is used to make copies of a strand of DNA. Although this test is accurate more quickly than the HIV antibody tests used more routinely, it is never 100 percent accurate. Also, the sperm count, motility, and percentage of normal forms in frozen samples are guaranteed to meet certain standards by many large sperm banks. With a fresh donor, such guarantees are impractical, since one needs to use the semen donated on the day of insemination.

DO SPERM DONORS TELL THE TRUTH?

Of course, couples using donor insemination usually are concerned about the donor. Couples often ask how the sperm bank knows the donor is telling the truth about his own life and his family medical history, particularly since he will be paid for his participation. Unfortunately, even the most careful sperm bank cannot guarantee that a donor is telling the complete truth. Sperm banks do not usually perform background checks on donors to look for a history of legal problems, but most do have extensive contacts with the donor over a number of months. To succeed as a semen donor, a man must be reliable enough to go through all required medical examinations, fill out extensive paperwork and questionnaires, and return time after time to donate semen (and samples have to be of repeated high quality, which requires abstaining from sex at regular times, too). Donors also have to return at least six months after their last sperm donation to be retested for STDs. One large sperm bank (California Cryobank) advertises on the Internet that they only accept 5 percent of donor applicants.

A few sperm banks have potential donors interviewed by a mental health professional or require that the donor complete a personality test that is interpreted by a psychologist. Such an evaluation does provide an extra way to assess the donor's motivation, honesty, and history of emotional problems.

HOW MUCH CAN WE FIND OUT ABOUT THE DONOR?

In past years, all couples knew about the donor was his coloring, physical build, ethnic background, and perhaps his occupation or major in college. Some couples still prefer to limit their information about the donor, perhaps because it helps them emotionally to minimize the influence of a third party in their family building. Not everyone wants to picture this stranger who will contribute the sperm cell for their baby. Increasingly, however, couples are interested in having more information about the donor. Many want to have a detailed medical history of the donor's family, in case their child develops a health problem in the future that could be genetic. Most sperm banks do offer such histories on their donors, typically including three generations of information. At least one sperm bank (Xytex) preserves genetic material from each donor so that genetic testing could be performed if necessary to diagnose or trace an inherited illness. This is an excellent practice, since the Human Genome Project will soon finish mapping all human genes, and the number of genetic tests available to diagnose disease or predict future disease risk is increasing with incredible speed.

Couples often prefer that the baby look something like the husband. Some sperm banks or Internet sites offer photographs of the donors, and one even offers his baby picture (Xytex)! Some offer to have one of their staff members match the donor by photo to the husband in the couple. In this way, the donor's privacy can be protected if he is not willing to have couples see his photograph. Of course, choosing a donor who looks like the husband is no guarantee that the child will resemble the husband's side of the family. A brown-haired, brown-eyed couple can have a blond, blue-eyed child if they had ancestors with fair coloring.

Other couples would like to choose a donor based on his intelligence, special talents, or personality. Some sperm banks will disclose a donor's Scholastic Aptitude Test (SAT) scores or college grade point average. Many will give information about whether the donor is a good athlete, musician, artist, and so on. Some describe the donor's personality, or have him write an essay about himself or record an audiotaped interview.

SPERM DONATION
AND THE PERFECT BABY

How useful is information about the donor's abilities or personality in predicting a child's traits? Intelligence, as measured by intelligence tests or achievement tests such as the SATs, is a reasonably good predictor of someone's performance in school. It is less successful at pinpointing who will succeed in life in terms of work achievements or family happiness. It is clear that genetics plays a strong role in intelligence, but both parents probably contribute a number of genes that play a role in learning abilities. It is also clear that the environment a child experiences has a strong influence on his or her future success. Knowing that a donor is a nuclear physicist may have some small value if you want a child who is a math whiz, but you also may be very disappointed to find your child has no special math or science abilities, regardless of the sperm that contributed to her or his heritage. Special talents in music or drawing also may run in families, but parents can give their child special training and exposure to music or art that is as crucial or more crucial than the genes the mother and the father contribute.

Research on personality shows that some very basic traits, such as shyness in new social situations or openness to trying new experiences, have some genetic basis. It is very difficult to trace a child's personality to the parents' dispositions, however. Even in an adult, psychological tests that measure personality only have very modest abilities to predict future behavior.

Even though it is not as feasible to create a designer baby as it might seem when you skim through a detailed catalog of sperm donors, the concept worries scholars who study the ethics of medical practice. It reminds them of *eugenics,* the attempt to breed human beings for desirable qualities. Eugenics has a long, dishonorable history in the 20th century. In the 1920s and 1930s, American scientists used poor research methods and even some faked data to try to prove that people who were not whites of northern European ancestry were inferior in intelligence. New emigrants to the United States were often labeled as mentally retarded, sometimes because they were given IQ tests when they could barely speak English. Some eugenicists rationalized that the poor or the disabled were genetically inferior, and unworthy of help from society, since governments should focus on survival of the fittest. This trend of thought peaked in the German Nazi era, when those labeled as genetically unfit, including Jews, gays, communists, political prisoners, and the disabled, were put to death.

Today, eugenics lives on as a philosophy, although it is often sugar-coated. In California, a sperm bank called the Repository for Germinal Choice offers sperm donors specially chosen for their intellectual achievements. This sperm bank began by trying to recruit Nobel laureates as donors. Not only were many unwilling to participate, but few of these elderly men had sperm with the high counts and motility needed to survive freezing and thawing well. Now the sperm bank uses professional journals to try to recruit young scientists as donors. Couples who want to use this sperm bank have to complete an application, demonstrating the mother's brightness and genetic fitness.

The web site for this sperm bank (http://www.alpha1net/~surrogate/sbank.html) states: "Humankind is far from perfect but can be improved gradually by increasing the proportion of advantageous genes in the human gene pool. The Repository provides one way to accomplish this." If you are considering becoming one of their customers, you must decide whether you agree philosophically with this concept.

DONOR INSEMINATION AROUND THE WORLD

It is interesting to compare the United States to other countries in terms of the practice and regulation of donor insemination. As we mentioned previously, the United States tends to allow public opinion and local laws to control infertility technology, whereas many European countries, such as England, France, Denmark, and Sweden, have national committees that create legal limitations on providing in vitro fertilization, donor insemination, and other controversial treatments.

In England, sperm donors can be paid a small sum for travel expenses, but not the larger amounts they would receive in the United States. France has outlawed payment of donors, as has Sweden. In Sweden, donors must be willing to participate in a national registry, and allow offspring at age 18 to find out their biological father's identity. At first this law led to a decrease in donor insemination, but more recently the available pool of donors has increased again. Swedish sperm donors recruited under the new law tend to be older and more altruistic than those in the United States. Donor insemination is banned in Muslim countries. In Israel, sperm banks operate under secular law, despite disapproval of the use of donor insemination by Orthodox Judaism. Many countries require signed consent of the husband and the wife for donor insemination, and only a few allow directed sperm donation.

DONOR INSEMINATION
VERSUS IVF-ICSI

Until recently, donor insemination was the only option besides adoption for couples with severe male infertility who wanted a child. Now that a majority of men with male factor infertility have a chance to have a genetic child by using IVF-ICSI, why choose donor insemination? We have studied this issue in our own patients. Some couples try IVF, but are unsuccessful in becoming pregnant. A few men also do not produce any live sperm cells in their testicles for use with IVF. Most couples who choose donor insemination as their first-line treatment, however, do so because IVF-ICSI is so expensive. Secondary concerns often mentioned are the limited success rates for IVF and the physical risks for the woman. In our program, most couples who chose donor insemination were clearly less well-off financially than couples who chose IVF-ICSI.

We have worried that couples who choose donor insemination primarily for financial reasons could feel resentful later that money got in the way of having a mutual genetic child. Will they treat their donor insemination child as second best? We doubt this will be a common problem, but the lack of insurance coverage for infertility treatment is a very real factor in couple's choices. Couples who choose donor insemination because it is affordable must look into their hearts and try to imagine whether they can value their child just as strongly as if he or she carried both of their genes.

Another reason to choose donor insemination over IVF-ICSI would be to avoid having a child with an inherited health problem. For example, a man who knew his genetic child would have a strong risk of a chronic childhood disease such as cystic fibrosis, or a disease that strikes in adulthood such as inherited colon cancer or Huntington's disease, might choose to have a child by using donor sperm. Our research suggests that only a few men consider donor insemination for such reasons. Couples are most likely to be concerned about a genetic risk if it could lead to mental retardation or death in childhood.

We and other infertility researchers have the impression that men who had biological children and then chose vasectomy are more accepting of donor insemination as an option than men who have had lifelong infertility and are childless. If a divorced or widowed man marries a younger woman and wants to start a second family, he may feel that donor insemination is an easier option than having a vasectomy reversal or having his wife undergo the risks of IVF-ICSI. Having a biological child may carry less weight in his decision, as he already has carried on his genetic heritage.

DONOR INSEMINATION
VERSUS ADOPTION

As we mentioned above, some couples choose adoption because of a fear that donor insemination is inherently unequal for the husband and the wife. With donor insemination, the wife gets a chance to have her own genetic child, carry a pregnancy, and give birth, but the husband has to parent a child not of his own blood. Couples may worry that the husband could not love another man's child, or that the child would be emotionally closer to the mother, with the father left out of the strong parental bonds.

On the other hand, couples often choose donor insemination over adoption precisely because the woman can contribute her genes and experience pregnancy and birth. They like the control they have over getting good prenatal care and the fact that the donor has been screened for health and other positive genetic qualities. The cost of donor insemination is far less than that of the great majority of adoptions. In fact, the financial difference between adoption and donor insemination is even greater than that between IVF-ICSI and donor insemination. If couples choose an anonymous donor, it is highly unlikely that he will ever appear on their doorstep, wanting to get to know his genetic offspring. Couples with infertility are often very concerned, in contrast, about birth parents wanting to reclaim an adopted child, or at least being an emotional competitor for love in their child's life in an open adoption. Couples may also like donor insemination because it avoids the intrusive home-study process. Last, but not least, there is no waiting list for donor insemination.

As fewer women have given up their children for adoption, many infertile couples perceive serious barriers to adopting. These include the very long delays in getting a child, concerns about the health of children whose parents may have used drugs or alcohol or have been HIV-positive, the negative way agencies may view parents who are over age 40 or not in perfect health, and the expense and uncertainties of international adoption.

On the other hand, adoption remains an act that is valued very positively by society, whereas donor insemination, rightly or wrongly, continues to carry some stigma. Couples who adopt have the satisfaction of knowing they are giving love and nurturance to a child who needed them. Couples who disclose using donor insemination may be told by friends or family that they are being selfish, or violating community or religious standards.

MEN'S AND WOMEN'S VIEWS ON DONOR INSEMINATION

Do men and women regard donor insemination differently? As we discuss in chapter 18, evolution may have sensitized men to resent bringing up children who are not their own biological offspring. In the general population, surveys suggest that men are more likely than women to reject the idea of having a child through donor insemination. When researchers asked the same questions of couples who had been treated for infertility, however, a similar (and larger) percentage of husbands and wives would consider using a donor to have a child. The experience of longing for a child changes some of the knee-jerk response to the idea of raising a child not biologically related to one parent. The same study found that better-educated couples were more likely to approve of donor insemination.

WOULD YOU BE ABLE
TO LOVE THE CHILD?

An extremely important question to consider in choosing donor insemination is whether both parents feel able to fully love and value the resulting child. More than anything, children need unconditional love and appreciation for their unique strengths. It is destructive to bring up a child and communicate a subtle message that he or she is not quite good enough. Luckily, it appears that couples who decide on donor insemination typically love their children very much. In fact, a study in four European countries comparing families with children aged four to eight conceived by donor insemination, born through IVF, adopted, or conceived without any infertility found that all of the parent groups who had confronted infertility rated parenting as less stressful and valued their children more than parents in the fertile group! Fathers spent more time with children in the post-infertility families and felt closer emotionally to their children. Those with children from donor insemination did not differ from those who had adopted or had their mutual genetic child by using IVF. The children were also rated as equally well-adjusted in the different family groupings. Most couples who use donor insemination are happily married and do not have a higher divorce rate than the general population after becoming parents.

When couples choosing donor insemination are studied over time, it is clear that they have the most doubts when they are deciding about it as an option. Once a pregnancy occurs, and even more once the baby is born, both partners feel more positive. Furthermore, wives tend to underestimate their husband's initial acceptance of donor insemination, while husbands see their wives as more gung ho than they actually are at first.

If you have doubts about your ability to love a child conceived with donor insemination, perhaps you can imagine the future by thinking about an experience of caring for a child who is not biologically related to you. Do you have any stepchildren? Have you ever been a teacher or a volunteer and become attached to one of your charges? Are you close to a niece or a nephew on your spouse's side of the family? Have you been a foster or an adoptive parent? A relationship with a child conceived via donor insemination is far less complicated than any of these situations because you and your spouse share the decision to conceive, the pregnancy, the birth, and all the parenting, without a birth parent, ex-spouse, or sibling in the picture.

VIEWS OF MAJOR RELIGIONS
ABOUT DONOR INSEMINATION

Donor insemination is not approved by a number of the world's religions. The table on the next page summarizes some beliefs about it.

SHOULD YOU CONSIDER A FRIEND
OR A FAMILY MEMBER AS DONOR?

A surprising number of couples with male factor infertility have thought about using a father, a brother, a cousin, or a good friend of the husband as a sperm donor. This may seem like a good way to at least have the child carry some genes from the father's family, or in the case of a friend, to know fully about the donor's background. Until very recently, any such arrangements were apt to be made between couple and donor without medical help, either collecting the donor's semen at home and using the old "turkey baster" technique to inseminate the wife, or in rare cases having the wife and the donor have intercourse. Since the use of known egg donors has become common, however, many infertility clinics are more willing to help a couple use a known semen donor.

If using a known donor, responsible physicians require that he be treated just like a donor at a sperm bank. He should be tested for sexually transmitted diseases such as HIV and hepatitis, provide a complete family health history, have genetic testing where appropriate, and have his semen frozen and be retested for HIV six months after the last sample is collected, before an insemination takes place.

Couple and donor should sit down with a mental health professional and discuss fully their expectations about the donor's relationship to the child, including whether the child will be told of its origins. If the donor is married, his wife should be a part of this process. Furthermore, an attorney should help the parties draw up a legal agreement in which the donor gives up parental rights to the child and the recipient couple assume them. In our experience, couples often back away from the idea of using a known donor when they realize how complicated it could

Religion	View on Donor Insemination	Reason for This View
Orthodox Judaism	Forbids donor insemination.	Since the child's father is unknown, incest could occur without the parties' realizing it. Some rabbis feel that using a non-Jewish donor avoids this concern. The donor is considered the legal father of the child.
Conservative or Reform Judaism	Rabbis' opinions may vary.	Same concerns as above.
Islam	Donor insemination is forbidden.	Donor insemination is considered adultery. It might lead to incest and also violates Islamic law by telling a lie about a child's genetic origins.
Catholicism	Donor insemination is not acceptable.	All conception should occur through sexual intercourse between two spouses, an act that symbolizes the sacred aspect of marriage. A child has a right to be born because of a holy act of marriage.
Protestant denominations	No official position on donor insemination.	Evangelical churches may be more likely to disapprove.

become. In a small study of known donors in New Zealand, 63 percent of couples planned to tell the child the identity of its biological father. Most felt the experience had made them feel closer to the donor, but about a fourth of the couples felt alienated from the donor over time.

> Leo had an aggressive type of testicular cancer at age 21 and had to endure months of chemotherapy. He also had an operation that left him unable to ejaculate semen. When he married at age 29, he and his wife agreed they would try for a child with donor insemination, since Leo's sperm count was still very low and IVF-ICSI was so expensive. Leo was in an unusual situation, however, because he had an identical twin, Larry. The infertility clinic pointed out that Larry, who never had testicular cancer, could easily donate sperm that would be genetically identical to Leo's. Leo rejected the idea, however. He and Larry had always resented the attention they received for being identical. Their mother had insisted on dressing them alike, and in their small community they had shared the same classrooms all through elementary school. The older they got, the more Leo and Larry drifted away from each other. As adults, they only saw each other at family gatherings, rarely seeking out each other's company for pleasure. In fact, they lived in different states. Leo adamantly rejected the idea of using Larry as a sperm donor, much preferring an anonymous donor from the sperm bank.

TO TELL OR NOT TO TELL?

One of the toughest emotional issues in donor insemination is whether to tell a child about its genetic parentage. Along with that decision come choices about telling family members or close friends about the child's origins. Until very recently, the great majority of people who used donated sperm were routinely counseled by their physicians to keep it a secret from the child and other family members.

Professionals' typical advice about secrecy has been changed by two trends in our society, however: open adoption policies and the use of donated oocytes (eggs). The great majority of adoptions in the United States used to be closed. The birth mother and adopting couple never knew each others' identities. Records were legally sealed. Until the 1950s or 1960s, adopting couples were also advised not to tell their children they were adopted. As adoption practices in the United States have changed, mental health professionals involved in adoption have taken a strong position that a child has a right to be informed about adoption as soon as he or she is old enough to understand. Many adoptions are now completely open, with birth mother and adopting parents meeting and even keeping some contact over the years. Despite the publicity about children of closed adoption seeking out their birth mothers, the great majority of adopted children make no attempt to find out about their genetic heritage. There is some evidence that open adoption leads to better psychological adjustment in families. Direct comparison studies with closed adoption are not possible, however, given the changes over the years in adoption policy.

Another influence toward openness with children has been the growing popularity of oocyte donation. By 1995, 8 percent of all assisted reproductive procedures in North America involved donated eggs. Because an egg donor must undergo an entire IVF stimulation cycle and egg retrieval, it is not easy to find women to volunteer, even with some payment for their time and trouble. Many clinics ask the infertile couple to bring their own donor, typically a relative or a close friend of the woman. In 1994, oocyte donation was offered by 163 clinics in the United States and Canada. Seventeen percent of donor egg cycles in 1994 used known donors. More families who use donated eggs plan to be open in telling the child about it, compared to families who use donated sperm. Perhaps this difference reflects more comfort among women compared to men in discussing their infertility or other family issues with friends. Egg donation is also a new procedure, begun in an era when in vitro fertilization is openly discussed on television and in magazines. Sperm donation began in an era when infertility was seen as a secret stigma.

The controversy about whether to tell a child about gamete donation remains, however, with passions running high on each side of the fence. Mental health professionals from the open adoption movement believe that no family should be allowed to conceive from donated gametes unless they plan to tell the child of his or her parentage. Furthermore, they would like to see an end to the practice of anonymous sperm or egg donation. They believe that secrets in a family are almost always destructive, and that a child born of confidential gamete donation will sense his or her lack of belonging to the family. Ultimately, they feel, a family member is likely to spill the beans in a way that will make the child feel rejected and unsure of his or her identity. Furthermore, many believe that each child has a right to know about his or her genetic heritage, and that lack of such knowledge will prevent a person from ever feeling whole.

We have little scientific evidence about whether knowledge of one's genetic heritage affects children's self-esteem or sense of identity, however. It is sobering to realize that if even 2 percent of people in the United States have been deceived about the identity of their biological father (the low end of the estimate of the rate of nonpaternity found in genetic testing performed to diagnose illness or for research), millions of Americans are living their lives with a false impression of their genetic background.

In studies of American and European married couples who have a child through sperm donation, at least two-thirds still believe that privacy about their decision is the best policy. Follow-ups of couples are also consistent in showing that of the parents who plan initially to be open, only a minority have told their offspring of their origins by middle childhood.

A common reason for choosing privacy with sperm donation is to protect the father's self-esteem. Many men do not want others to know about their infertility. Fathers also express fear that the child will love them less, knowing about the lack of a genetic connection. As we mentioned previously, the use of donated sperm or eggs also is disapproved by several major religions. Parents may legitimately worry that their child will be rejected by family members or stigmatized in social situations, if his or her origins are known. Since most donors in the United States are anonymous, couples wonder if it is worth telling a child about the genetic parent. Unless they have used one of the few sperm banks that offer identified donors, they are only likely to know the donor's coloring, education, profession, and ethnic group. This lack of information could frustrate a child who knew about the donation and wanted detailed facts about his or her genetic heritage.

It is difficult to study the impact of privacy on the children of donated gametes because the great majority of families successfully conceal their story, unless forced to reveal it by a rare medical emergency, such as the need for a bone marrow transplant. The follow-up studies that have been published are based on families who have not told their children of their origins, yet no obvious ill effects are seen. Unfortunately, the media loves to focus on the rare situations in which children find out about donor insemination in some traumatic way; for example, when the father in the family seeks a divorce and overtly rejects the child. A recent news story featured interviews with three donor offspring who wanted to find their genetic fathers and felt their identities were incomplete without knowing the men involved. These stories are obviously not the typical experience of the hundreds of thousands of children born from donor insemination.

Couples who think they would like to tell their child about using a donor should seriously consider using one of the sperm banks that has donors willing to meet their offspring as adults, or who at least fill out a detailed questionnaire on their backgrounds that recipient families can keep.

Another issue to keep in mind is the growing amount of genetic information being used in medicine. It probably will not be many years before young people are routinely tested for genes that can identify their later risk of breast cancer or heart disease. Then preventive lifestyle changes or medications could be used to reduce disease risks. If physicians depend on family medical histories to decide what genetic tests to order, a child may be at a disadvantage if her or his true genetic profile is unknown. Increased use of genetic testing and information in the future also may make it more difficult to keep donor insemination a secret. One of us recently heard of a high school biology class that planned a project on DNA fingerprinting for each student. Nowadays parents feel their child is unlikely to find out about donor insemination if the father and donor match in ethnicity, physical traits, and blood type. In the future, that may not be enough.

WHEN AND HOW TO TELL A CHILD

If you choose to tell your child about donor insemination, when and how should you do it? Again, the research we have available provides little guidance. The adoption model suggests using stories and books to tell the child starting in the toddler years. Donor insemination is a bit complicated, however. To understand the concept, a child must be able to comprehend that babies come from a sperm and an egg uniting. Although a couple of storybooks on donor insemination manage to present this information without mentioning genitals or sex at all (see "Resources"), most three- or four-year-olds are going to be curious about how these eggs and sperm usually manage to get together! Thus talking about donor insemination means having the dreaded birds and bees conversation. Perhaps this is one reason that even parents who intend to tell their children typically never find a comfortable time. We would encourage all parents to give children age-appropriate, accurate information about sexuality, however.

Some recent research on children's understanding of why offspring resemble their parents suggests that most are unable to really comprehend the idea of physical heredity until they are about seven years old. Younger children did not know that a baby would resemble its birth parents physically, and its adoptive parents in terms of beliefs. Of course, many of these children were also not familiar with the facts of reproduction, and a bright child might well be able to understand the idea of donor insemination after a simple explanation about conception and birth. It is probably best to tell children about donor insemination before they reach adolescence. A teenager could feel shocked and insecure about such an unexpected revelation during a crucial time in the development of adult identity and emotional independence from the family.

Perhaps the most important element of the story should be the parents' strong wish for a child and joy at finally having a baby. A child should never be told about donor insemination as a rationale for one parent's neglectful treatment, as a way of winning points in a marital battle, or in a moment of anger.

MAKING A BALANCED DECISION

We believe that parents can do an excellent job of raising their child no matter which choice they make. Indeed, a recent study of donor insemination families found that the decision whether to tell the child about its origins bore no relationship to the parents' bonding with the child. Parents who conceive a child through donor gametes should think about the attitude in their family and community toward nontraditional families. A couple with a close-knit family with very traditional values or who lives in a small community with conservative views about gamete donation may have valid fears about their child being rejected or ostracized.

If the plan is to keep the use of donor gametes a secret from the child, ideally nobody else should be told, including the couple's parents, siblings, or friends. When someone else knows about the donation, the parents are no longer completely in control of whether the child is told. One recent study found that about 60 percent of couples who conceived a child through sperm donation had told someone about their decision. Eighty percent of these couples, however, regretted having told and would not tell anyone about the procedure if they could go back and make the decision again. The more people a couple told about sperm donation, the more likely they were later to regret having told anyone. These regrets stemmed from the feeling that now they had no choice about whether to reveal the story to their child. Even if a couple plans to be open with their child, it may be wise to confide only in close friends and family members whose support and caring can be trusted.

It is crucial that husband and wife agree on how to handle confidentiality. At every step of the way, from the decision to use a donor, through the pregnancy, and after a child is born, the parents must communicate openly with each other about what to tell the child.

The crucial task of parenting is to help a child feel loved and valued for his or her unique strengths. This is a central challenge for all parents, whether we contribute to our child's genes or not. Even a genetic child is far from an exact combination of the parents. Differences and diverse talents should be recognized and enjoyed.

By now readers should have a clear grasp of the medical aspects of male infertility and its treatments. We devote Part Three of this book to the emotional issues involved in coping with a diagnosis of male infertility, including the man's versus the woman's point of view, how to pull together as a team, understanding spiritual concerns, and untangling your finances to pay for infertility treatment. We also describe how couples tackle decisions such as whether to adopt or to remain without children.

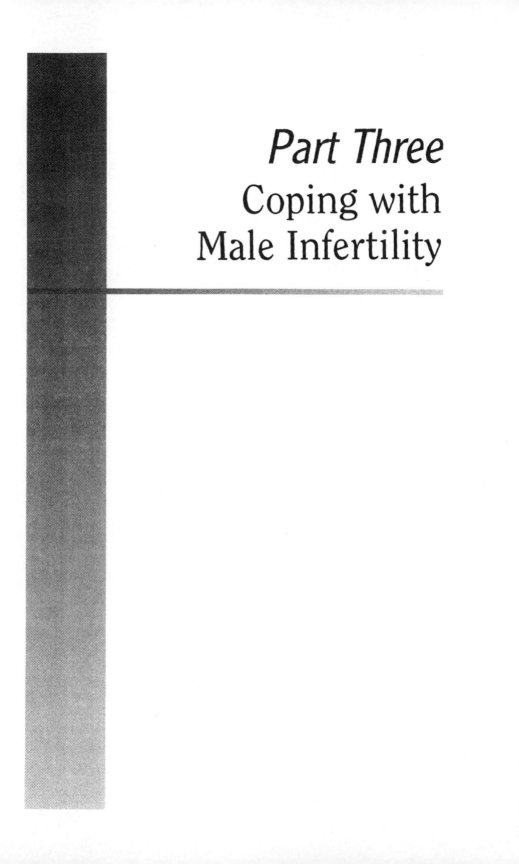

Part Three
Coping with Male Infertility

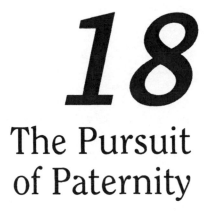

The Pursuit
of Paternity

Why do men want to have children? Possible motives include the wish to continue your family line and name; to fulfill a religious or spiritual commitment to future generations; to pass on qualities in yourself that you think are valuable to society; to express the love you feel for your wife; to give her the experience of pregnancy and motherhood; to experience the joys and sorrows of raising a child; to share parenthood with your mate as a team; to give your child all the chances and more that your parents gave you; to have someone to care about you and for you in your old age; to feel that you are fully an adult; or to show the world that you are able to be a father.

Modern science, medicine, and philosophy offer a variety of perspectives on the meaning of parenthood. Several will be highlighted in this chapter. Our goal is to give you a chance to look at these different points of view, and compare them with your own feelings and beliefs about being a parent. Understanding your own motives for having children can help you make some of the difficult choices that infertility brings: whether to gamble your money and energy on surgery that may improve your chances of a pregnancy or on assisted reproductive techniques, whether to consider adoption or donor insemination, or if you should resign yourself to living without children.

IDEAS FROM
EVOLUTIONARY BIOLOGY

A central idea in sociobiology is that each animal, or human, has a degree of *reproductive fitness.* (Sociobiologists are scientists who study how evolution has shaped the behavior of animals and humans.) You cannot increase your reproductive fitness by working out at the gym or taking vitamins. As it turns out, it depends on the number of grandchildren you have. Those men and women who have the most descendants win the evolutionary lottery. Their genes will help to determine the future direction of humankind. This process is far from random. Sociobiologists believe that our mating styles have been shaped by millions of years of evolution to maximize our chances of having offspring. After all, we are our ancestors' success stories. Sociobiologists also believe that human men and women have different styles of mating. This is called the theory of *parental investment.*

WOMEN SHOULD
MAKE SMART CHOICES

A human mother can only produce a very few children in her lifetime. Pregnancy consumes time and physical energy. Since evolution is a slow process, humans were shaped by their lives in nomadic bands of hunters and gatherers, the norm until about 10,000 years ago, when farming was invented. In the hunting and gathering peoples remaining today, a woman only bears a child on the average of once every four years. She spends the next several years breast-feeding (which prevents another pregnancy) and toting around that baby, providing almost all of its nutrition and protecting it from harm. In these conditions, without modern nutrition and medicine, a woman's reproductive years probably only last from about age 18 until 30 or so. If one of her children dies, or grows up to be an unhealthy, undesirable mate, her reproductive fitness (e.g., her contribution to future generations) is very much at risk.

Thus, for our ancestral mother, the best strategy to have a healthy child was to pick a father for her children who had the best possible genes to contribute—a strong, healthy man. In addition, her children would have a much better chance of survival if their father stuck around to contribute to raising them. Of course, the most reliable family man was not always the best genetic specimen. Thus another pattern to increase a woman's reproductive fitness might be to get pregnant secretly with the most genetically desirable man around, but let her mate think the baby was really his own. A woman who wanted to deceive her husband would have an advantage over her primate cousins, like chimpanzees or gorillas. The females of those species broadcast that they are in a fertile period through visible swellings or color changes in their genitals. In humans, ovulation is hidden; that is, the woman's body does not signal her fertile time to the man. Unlike most other primates who solicit sex mainly at ovulation, human women feel desire for sex at a fairly constant level throughout the menstrual cycle. Women are often aware of their own ovulation, however, because they feel soreness in the area of the ovaries or see an increase in clear vaginal discharge. Studies suggest that, whether women are conscious of it or not, most acts of female infidelity occur during peak fertility times. Anthropologists also find that practically every society includes women and men who are unfaithful to their mates.

ARE MEN PROGRAMMED TO SOW WILD OATS?

Infidelity is even more advantageous for men than for women, according to sociobiology. A man does not have to spend nine months of his life to create a child. All it takes is one ejaculation. A man who fathers many children with a variety of women has the greatest chance of keeping his genes in the pool. Of course, a father's care also makes an important contribution to a child's survival, and a man who fathers many children cannot nurture them all, unless he is, for example, a sultan with a harem and vast riches. In many human cultures that have been studied, wealthy and powerful men are allowed to have more than one wife. For the ordinary man in the street, however, the best strategy might be stealth. If he can have a small family of his own, his reproductive fitness will be about average. If he also gets another man's wife pregnant, however, and she deceives her husband into raising the baby as his own, the lover's reproductive success will soar without much investment on his own part.

PATERNITY:
THE PRIZE IN THE WAR OF THE SEXES

Sociobiology provides a rationale for the war between the sexes. Women have the power to deceive men about paternity. Sociobiologists would say that double standards about sexual freedom for men and women are based in our biology. Cultural and religious traditions that prize virginity and fidelity in women arose from eons of evolution, shaping men to control women's sexuality and to ensure that the children they raise will carry their own genes. In most cultures around the world, adultery on a woman's part is punished severely while male infidelity is considered a minor violation. The double standard only grew stronger as agriculture developed and then city life began. Paternity defined how property was inherited, with land and money passed from father to son. In ancient Rome, children were actually legally the property of their father.

A SOCIOBIOLOGICAL VIEW
OF MALE INFERTILITY

What does sociobiology have to do with a man's feelings on finding out he has a problem with fertility? One perspective is that his emotional reaction is not only based on his life experience and circumstances, but on his inherited drive to reproduce himself. From our experience over the years, we think men are less accepting than women of children not genetically related. Of course there are exceptions, but as a rule, men have more difficulty adjusting to the idea of parenting a child born from donor insemination than women do with egg donation. Men are also less open to the idea of adoption and more ready to accept living without children. An exception, as we have mentioned before, is the older man who had several children and then had a vasectomy. He may not care as much whether the baby he raises with a new wife is genetically related to him. The sociobiologist would say that he is already confident that he has fulfilled his reproductive potential.

Although raising a child that is not genetically hers also does not help a woman's reproductive fitness, women have not had to worry about being deceived about their genetic link with their children. Also, motherhood is a more central part of a woman's role in most cultures than fatherhood is to men.

Derek was 32 and married for three years when he and his wife, Melinda, sought help for infertility. Everything checked out normal on her side, but Derek was found to have no sperm in his semen. Further tests showed that he had been born without a vas deferens. Derek was found to have two mutations in the gene associated with cystic fibrosis. Melinda also went through genetic testing, and luckily was found not to have a mutation in her parallel genes. Still, given limitations in the genetic testing, the couple was given a 1 in 400 chance that their mutual child could be born with cystic fibrosis. Their options were to have sperm cells retrieved from Derek's testicles and use these for in vitro fertilization with intracytoplasmic sperm injection (IVF-ICSI), to have Melinda undergo insemination from a donor, or to adopt a child.

Melinda was leaning toward donor insemination, at least to have a first baby. It was the fastest and least expensive option. She wanted to be a mother as soon as possible and worried about the small risk of cystic fibrosis, especially since she did not believe she could terminate a pregnancy if prenatal testing showed that the baby would have the illness. Derek felt strongly that they should start with IVF, however. If it failed, he was willing to adopt, but he did not think he could love a child born from donor insemination. "It wouldn't be fair," he said, "because Melinda would be the real mother, but I wouldn't be the real father. I think the child would be closer to her, and I'd feel left out. The bottom line is that I can't deal with Melinda having some other guy's baby." The couple proceeded with IVF and were successful on their second try. Melinda was frequently irritable with the side effects, and the couple had a major blowup when the first cycle failed. Both felt afterward that the infertility experience had strained their relationship.

It is uncomfortable to think that feelings like Derek's—and our own—are somehow the product of biology rather than free will. Paternity is a complex issue, and sociobiology is only a group of theories, and ones that are often hard to prove, especially for humans. Given the common patterns of gender relationships in societies around the world, however, it is hard to dismiss sociobiology as an explanation for some of our motives about parenthood.

AN ETHICAL OR SPIRITUAL PERSPECTIVE:
BIOLOGY IS NOT DESTINY

Another way to look at parenthood is to think of the ethical or moral val-ues of our own culture. A well-known bioethicist, Dr. Thomas Murray, recently published a book of essays called *The Worth of the Child.* He believes that we regard children differently than in the past. Not only do we no longer view a son or daughter as property, we have also gone beyond the view that a parent's main obligation is to fill a child's belly and make sure it has clothes, education, and a place to live. Modern par-ent-child relationships are ideally based on mutual love and trust. Murray believes that good parents love their children unconditionally, not expecting them to be perfect.

A shift in the way we value children can also be seen in the elimina-tion of child labor in modern, industrialized nations, giving kids many years to play and learn. A parallel change has happened in the way we discipline our children, so that the "good whipping" of a past generation would be seen as child abuse today.

If we look at parenthood from this vantage, contributing a sperm is only a tiny part of the package. It is the years of nurturing a child that make a man (or a woman) a parent. Whether the child is one's own, a stepchild, an adopted child, or a child born from donor insemination, each is a uniquely valuable human being in need of love and care. The sadness of infertility certainly includes giving up the dream of seeing one's own features blended with your beloved's in a new, tiny face. It also is the grief of breaking the chain that connects you with your known family and those unknowable ancestors whose genes fill up your chro-mosomes. But being infertile does not have to mean giving up being a father.

SPECIAL ISSUES FOR MEN
IN COPING WITH INFERTILITY

Infertility is clearly a major stress for most men, just as it is for women. Our society's expectations for men can make it difficult to sort out the emotions that infertility brings.

• Men often believe they should keep their feelings of sadness inside. If you do not express your grief about infertility, your partner and family may not realize how much you are hurting. It can be healthy to talk to one or two people you trust, or even to allow yourself to cry.

- Women typically talk about their emotional stresses with other women—mother, sisters, or friends. Men are more likely to share enjoyable activities with male family or friends. Men discuss successes with other men, but not problems. This can leave a man who has infertility feeling isolated. If you do not have a father, a brother, or a friend who you think would understand your feelings about infertility, perhaps you could use the infertility sites on the Internet (see "Resources") to read other men's comments or to participate in a bulletin board or a chat room.

- Some men had very fulfilling and loving relationships with their own fathers, and would like to re-create similar bonds with their own children. Other men never felt close to their fathers and would like to be a warmer and more involved dad with their future children. Thinking back on your experiences with your own father may help you sort out some of your feelings about having a biological child or pursuing parenthood through donor insemination or adoption.

This chapter discussed some special issues that may affect men's attitudes toward fatherhood. Next we look at the unique point of view that women have when in a relationship confronting male infertility.

19

The Female Side
of Male Infertility

This chapter is written especially for the wife or the female partner of the man with infertility, but men may also want to read it for some insight into the female perspective. Our years of experience with infertility have convinced us that men and women cope differently with the emotions the problem brings.

GENDER AND
EMOTIONAL COPING STYLES

A series of popular self-help books suggest that men and women deal with emotion so differently that they seem to be from different planets. Although this is an exaggeration, infertility often highlights gender differences in coping. A variety of research studies have found that within an infertile couple, the wife is typically more emotionally distressed than the husband. When couples fail to conceive through in vitro fertilization (IVF), both partners are disappointed and sad, but more women than men become significantly depressed.

Why do men report less desperation about infertility? Our culture teaches men to cope with stress by solving problems rather than by expressing emotion. The ideal for a man is to confront a stress head-on, figure out what to do about it, and then finish the job. In contrast, women are encouraged to focus on their emotions and relationships with others. Women have much more social permission than men to acknowledge sadness, fear, or self-doubts. When a woman gets the news that she has a physical problem getting pregnant, having a good cry often relieves some of her stress. A man who lets himself cry at the news of an abnormal sperm count may just feel worse, as if he is being weak. Whereas women torture themselves with guilt and grief, men typically feel shame, humiliation, and anger. Men take Viagra and women take Prozac. If you take our stereotype of the male role to its extreme, an infertile man may not only see himself as failing to be a good provider to his wife who wants a child, he may feel he does not even qualify as a real man.

Despite feminism and the large number of women who work outside the home, being a mother is still a more central part of our cultural ideal for women than being a father is for men. For women, it is not only crucial to get pregnant and give birth, but to have a lifelong commitment to raising children. Images of men in the media and popular culture focus more on the physical ability to father a pregnancy and less on success in nurturing children. As one of our patients said recently, "When the guys get together, they joke about whether their sperm are good swimmers. They don't know about my problem, but inside I really feel lousy, like I don't measure up."

This brings up another point: women typically get a good deal of comfort from discussing their battle with infertility with friends and family. Men, in contrast, often feel very private about infertility, particularly when the medical problem is on the male side, and are upset if a wife or a partner discloses the problem to others. Male friends or kin are much less likely than women to discuss infertility openly. Some men actually experience taunting from others at work if word of their problem gets out. Male infertility is often seen as a clue that a man is not performing well sexually—a connection not typically made for women.

BRIDGING THE GENDER GAP

If you are a woman who knows or suspects that your partner has a male infertility problem, you may be reading this book to figure out:

- Whether he really wants a child as much as you do
- How to get him to go to the doctor and get infertility treatment rolling

- How to get him to talk to you about his feelings
- How to get the emotional support you need without violating his need for privacy about the infertility

Let's look at each of these issues in turn.

Does He Want a Baby As Much As You Do?   This is a dangerous question to ponder. If you believe your mate does not want a baby as much as you, you will probably feel resentful and disappointed. It is more likely that he wants a baby in a different way. You may have a desperate emotional yearning to hold your own baby in your arms. He may dream more abstractly about sharing Little League or seeing a child graduate from college. As we mentioned earlier, men also may not express their negative feelings, such as grief or anxiety about infertility, because they have been indoctrinated to be logical.

There are several reasons why women often feel more distress than men about infertility, however. As a woman, you experience a direct confrontation with infertility each month when you get your period, an event that tends to sharpen and focus your sadness about not conceiving. Women are also more likely than men to modify career goals in the expectation of staying home full-time or part-time with a new baby. Uncertainty about when or whether a pregnancy will occur often causes women to feel burnout at work. In contrast, men's jobs are more likely to provide a welcome distraction from worrying about having children. Men also are more free of the infamous biological clock that limits women's childbearing years.

In our society, women tend to marry older men. With the increase in divorce rates to around 50 percent of all marriages, some women end up with a man who has already had children. In infertility clinics we are likely to see couples in which the husband had a vasectomy, thinking he was finished with his family. Here is a typical story.

> Dan was an athletic and young-looking company president of 50, married to Tammy, a 35-year-old personnel consultant. Dan had three sons, aged 22, 18, and 16. Tammy had also had a brief first marriage, but had only been pregnant once at age 19, when she chose to have an abortion rather than have to drop out of college. Dan had been divorced for several years when he and Tammy met. Over their dating, she developed a cordial relationship with his younger two sons, who usually spent weekends with their father. When Dan asked Tammy to marry him, he offered to have his

vasectomy surgically reversed so that the couple could have a child together. She happily agreed to this plan.

Unfortunately, the vasectomy reversal was not successful and after two years of repeated semen analyses, Dan's urologist advised the couple to either try in vitro fertilization with intracytoplasmic sperm injection (IVF-ICSI), a technique that bypasses low sperm counts and motility by injecting a sperm cell directly into each egg, or to consider using semen from a donor to become pregnant. Dan told Tammy that the choice was up to her. They could afford the money for IVF, but he worried about the health risks for Tammy, whose fertility appeared to be normal. He felt he could love the child even if he was not the biological father. It was Tammy who cared enough about having Dan's genetic child to choose IVF over donor insemination.

Does Dan feel as strongly about having a child as Tammy does? Probably not, since he has already had the experience of being a parent. Yet he is ready to do all he can to create a child, and to love that child without reserve. In other couples with a similar history, the husband may refuse to consider having a child, giving the woman the ultimatum of accepting childlessness as a condition of staying married. Less extreme, but not uncommon, is the husband agreeing to have one more child, but telling his wife that she must do the lion's share of the work of parenting. It is best if couples have discussed these issues thoroughly before they marry, but sometimes a woman thinks she can live without being a mother, only to find when her biological clock is running out that she longs desperately for a baby.

Each partner in the couple does not need to start out with the same exact amount of need or type of motivation to have a baby. They do need a shared vision, however, of how parenthood will change their lives and their relationship. Men often find they love their babies more easily and naturally than they imagined they could. A man who is adamant that he does not want a baby, however, is not a good candidate for fatherhood. Furthermore, having a baby is not a good strategy for strengthening a relationship that is already very fragile.

How Can You Get Him to Go to the Doctor?   Since male causes for infertility are about as common as female factors, and getting a semen sample is relatively inexpensive and not physically painful, a semen analysis should be one of the first tests ordered when a physician is trying to find out why a woman is not getting pregnant. Some men do not try to prevent their wives from undergoing much more expensive and risky examinations, like a *hysterosalpingogram* (a test in which X-ray dye is injected into the uterus so that its interior and the fallopian tubes can be seen) or a laparoscopy (a minor surgery using an optical scope to examine the pelvic cavity and its organs), but refuse to see a doctor themselves. We know that men, in general, are less apt to seek medical care or take preventive health measures, such as wearing seat belts or sunscreen, than women. A young man who has never had a major health problem does not have the expectation of a routine, yearly medical examination as most women do with their gynecologists. Men also are more likely than women to cope with a health threat by avoiding the whole situation. On the surface, the problem may seem to be procrastination—he is always too busy to make the doctor's appointment, although he manages to work overtime, play tennis, and spend hours on the Internet. In reality, he may not wish to confront the possibility that he could be the one who is infertile.

If your partner is holding up the infertility evaluation, tell him clearly how important having a baby is to you. Try asking in an assertive and positive way for him to be half of the team in solving this problem. Let him know you will not love or value him less if he does not have a good sperm count, just as you expect he will continue to feel committed to you if the infertility is related to your medical problems. If you think the dread of giving a semen sample is holding him back, ask him to read chapter 3 of this book. *Avoid making threats to leave the marriage if he does not participate in the evaluation.* You do not want to create a "shotgun" baby, but rather to share the decision to try for a pregnancy out of your love for each other and wish for a family. If you are seriously considering divorce, you are not in a good place to start the struggle with infertility treatment.

Getting Your Man to Wear His Heart on His Sleeve.   Volumes have been written (mostly by women) about how to get men to recognize and disclose their inner emotions. Maybe your husband is a postmodern kind of guy, and can tell you what he is thinking and feeling, or cry without shame. Many men, however, react to a diagnosis of male infertility with stony silence followed either by repeated attempts to avoid the topic, or a concentrated effort to solve the problem medically. If a man copes by trying hard to ignore his feelings, he may also have trouble being supportive when you express your emotions. If you cry when you get your period, your husband may react by trying to cheer you up or hush you up. He also may get exasperated if you do not want to attend a family baby shower or a holiday party where babies will be shown off. His lack of empathy may just make you feel more guilty and upset.

It is usually best if you do not pressure your partner to express emotions. Recognize that you and he have different ways of coping with the infertility. Neither is right or wrong per se. Let him know what he could do to be more supportive to you, however, such as holding you in his arms when you are sad, or making a helpful comment such as, "I know how you feel. It is okay to cry." He could also give you extra support when you need to attend family occasions where pregnant relatives or infants will be present, or at least be understanding if you feel you cannot bear to go.

Finding Emotional Support without Violating His Privacy.   Very commonly, women going through infertility treatment have a need to talk over their feelings and experiences with a close friend, a sister, or mother. Men, in contrast, may not want anyone to know about their problem and do not understand why the wife would need to talk about it. Given that many men do not cope by sharing feelings, the husband's need for privacy leaves the wife without an outlet for emotional support. Sometimes these gender roles are reversed, however.

If you are both very open in discussing your attempts to have children, no problem exists. If you both share a preference for privacy, the main issue is making sure you present a united front when friends or family members ask about your plans for parenthood. If you disagree on who and how much to tell, you need a verbal contract with each other. If one partner feels it would be humiliating or painful for anyone in your family or social circle to know about the problem, the partner who needs some emotional support and sharing can consider:

- Talking individually to a mental health professional familiar with infertility. Then your confidentiality is assured and you can get expert advice on coping.

- Attending a support group for people with infertility; for example, through Resolve (see "Resources") or your local infertility clinic. Make sure, however, that the group does not include anyone you know, and that the ground rules of the group are to keep each other's stories and names confidential.

- Exchanging information via the Internet on your computer with other couples experiencing infertility (see "Resources").

Alternatively, the more private partner may be able to tolerate one or several people knowing about the problem. It is very important to specify, however, who can be told, and how much information can be shared. Remember that when considering long-term privacy about a treatment, particularly using donor insemination without telling the child about it, you may be better off not informing anyone who could later violate your confidence (see chapter 17).

> Alfredo and Rosa had just gotten pregnant using semen from an anonymous donor. They had previously been through two cycles of IVF without a pregnancy. Their families both were Catholic, first-generation immigrants from Mexico, and they believed their parents would disapprove of their choice, perhaps even reject their child. They also lived in a small town where Alfredo was fire chief and Rosa was an elementary school teacher. They did not want gossip about his fertility going around. They had not even told their parish priest about their treatments, again fearing he would take a disapproving stance. They had agreed never to tell their child about the donor insemination unless some rare medical emergency made it necessary. Still, Rosa worried about whether the family secret would somehow damage their child, and wished she could talk to someone else who had made the same choice. She posted some of her concerns anonymously on an Internet site for couples with infertility. She got responses from two women who had already had babies through donor insemination, and would correspond with her. Just knowing that other families had coped with the same situation helped Rosa get through her pregnancy with less anxiety. Alfredo also ended up having some dialogue with one of the husbands. The couples all agreed not to exchange their names or addresses so that everyone could remain comfortable about privacy.

WHY CAN'T A MAN
BE MORE LIKE A WOMAN?

Until very recent times, men lamented that women were ruled by their hormones, unfit to make important decisions, and mainly useful for reproductive purposes (i.e., sex and motherhood). With changing values about men's and women's roles, the tables have been turned. Women are wondering why their men cannot escape the confines of the traditional male role and act more like their girlfriends—admit their fears and worries, confess to their failures, and share a good cry. Gender roles have not changed that radically for most couples, however. You can promote some compromise in your relationship. Maybe you can have your menstrual cries alone in the bedroom, or your husband can tell his best friend about going through IVF. It is most important, however, that you each try to understand and respect the other's different ways of coping with infertility and become—as we suggest in the next chapter—a team.

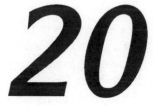

Coping with Infertility as a Team

Whether medical problems interfering with fertility are discovered only in the male partner of a couple or in both partners, infertility is a joint problem. You are having trouble as a couple getting pregnant, so it is crucial that you see yourselves as a team in coping with infertility. A majority of couples actually say that infertility has brought them closer together, particularly if they were already good at communicating. Only a minority of couples find that infertility threatens their love for one another. Nevertheless, even a couple with a happy relationship will confront stressful issues during infertility treatment. This chapter suggests some strategies to increase a couple's solidarity as they try to conceive.

AVOIDING BLAME

When diagnostic tests uncover the cause or causes of infertility, it is typical that the partner labeled with a problem feels not only distress for his or her own imperfection, but also guilt at the prospect of depriving the spouse of the joys of parenthood. It may be easier when the fertility problem was known to both partners before they committed to their relationship, since decisions about how or whether to have a child are usually discussed then and both partners take responsibility for their choices. More commonly, problems with fertility only become apparent after some time of trying for a pregnancy.

The 20 percent of infertile couples in which both partners are identified as having medical problems may have the easiest time adjusting, since neither spouse feels totally at fault. When only the husband has been diagnosed with a problem, however, a number of men have told us they felt so upset that they offered their wife a divorce so that she could marry someone who could give her children. Very few women accept such an offer, and fortunately, most men are able let go of their sense of shame and focus, instead, on solving the problem of infertility.

Occasionally we also see couples in which the wife does blame her husband for the infertility, and takes out her anger on him. She may belittle him, discuss his infertility with friends and family against his wishes, or even have an extramarital affair (sometimes to demonstrate that she can get pregnant). Such a lack of empathy may signal a need for counseling on the wife's part, or for both partners, since such behavior often is a sign that anger has built up over the years about other marital issues.

One of the frustrations of infertility is that there is rarely any way it could have been prevented. Sometimes, however, you need to come to terms with regrets about past choices. An example is when infertility results from a sexually transmitted disease (STD) (see chapter 9). Many young people experiment with sexual relationships before marriage, and all it takes is one infected partner. Nobody catches an STD on purpose. A choice to have a vasectomy is another example. As much as the man may regret his sterilization when he decides he would like to have another child, he cannot undo the past. When he had the original surgery, he was responding to a different set of circumstances. A decision to put off trying for a pregnancy also may seem foolish in retrospect. Sometimes one partner blames the other for delaying attempts to conceive a child until the woman's fertility had started to decline. Hindsight is always 20/20, but holding on to guilt about past choices will only make you miserable.

If you find yourself unable to let go of blame, whether self-blame or anger at your partner, you may want to speak with a mental health professional. You may want to find a new way to talk to yourself about the problem. For example, instead of telling yourself, "I am not a real man because I cannot give my wife a child," you could practice the thoughts, "I am a good husband in all sorts of ways. I am doing my best to work with my wife to find a way to be a parent. If she were the one with the medical infertility problem, I would not love her any less."

Spouses can help each other to change patterns of thinking and feeling by refusing to accept blaming statements and finding a different perspective on the problem. For example, if a husband tells his wife, "I am not good enough for you, because I can't make you pregnant," she can respond, "I value you for all the good things you bring to our marriage. I am sad that we are having trouble having a baby, but that does not make me love or value you less."

SHOWING SUPPORT

In the course of infertility treatment, there are typically many anxious and sad moments, such as anticipating uncomfortable medical tests or procedures, waiting for test results, finding out that a pregnancy has not occurred, or enduring a miscarriage. Partners need ways to show emotional support for each other at these times. As we discussed in the previous chapter, it is common for women to want to talk about their fears or to cry, whereas men often cope by trying to stay logical, and stick to the facts. Confronted by a wife's shakiness or tears, a man may be unsure how to help. He may try to cheer her up or, if that does not work, leave the scene. A more helpful tactic is to sit down, give your wife a hug, and tell her you love her and are sorry she is feeling so bad. You do not have to fix the situation, just let her know that you understand.

Women often make the mistake of trying to get a man to talk it out when he is giving signals that he is not ready. Pushing a man to show feelings may backfire, making him angry and defensive. Give him some space to react emotionally to bad news. Then find a relaxed and private time and place to talk. Realize that while you may feel it would be healthy to open up about emotions, men often cope effectively with infertility by focusing on problem solving rather than feelings.

If one partner, typically the wife, is so sad about infertility that it is difficult to go to events such as baby showers or child-centered holiday parties, the other spouse should try to understand. Even if you do not share the feeling, your spouse has a right to her or his own emotional reaction. Again, the two of you may be able to compromise—for example, to go to a holiday lunch with the family, but only stay for a couple of hours, or to arrange a signal that your spouse can give you if she or he needs extra attention or support, or is just feeling a strong need to leave.

SHARING DECISIONS
ABOUT TREATMENT OPTIONS

When a couple is given choices between treatment options—for example, using in vitro fertilization with intracytoplasmic sperm injection (IVF-ICSI), donor insemination, adoption, or remaining childless—partners often have different initial reactions or priorities. Considerations include difficult issues such as whether to gamble large amounts of money on treatments with limited success rates, or to give up the dream of a mutual, genetic child. If you and your partner find yourself having different opinions about what to do next, you need to reach a livable compromise. If issues relating to religion or ethics are complicating things, you may want to find a bioethicist (a specialist in medical ethics, often employed by a large hospital or a medical school) or a member of your clergy who can help you examine your spiritual beliefs (see chapter 22). If it is difficult for spouses to negotiate with each other, a mental health professional familiar with infertility issues can help you discuss your concerns calmly, highlighting areas of anxiety and also of agreement.

Some particularly important points to keep in mind:

- One partner should never make a unilateral decision about infertility treatment options. For example, a wife should never try to deceive her husband by seeking donor insemination without his knowledge and consent. By the same token, it will have a negative impact on a marriage if the wife very much wants to try in vitro fertilization (IVF) and the husband will not even consider or discuss spending the money to do so.

- One partner should never use an ultimatum about divorce to coerce the other into trying a particular infertility treatment. We have seen this tactic backfire too many times.

THE PARADOX OF IVF-ICSI

With the success of IVF-ICSI in helping couples with severe male infertility conceive, a paradox also occurs. It is typically the man in the couple who has the major infertility problem, but it is the woman who must undergo the hassles and risks of an IVF hormonal stimulation cycle and egg retrieval (although the husband may also have minor surgery to retrieve sperm cells). If the couple chooses donor insemination instead, the wife has a much easier role, yet will still get to have a child that carries her genes. Many women say they are willing to endure an IVF cycle to have a chance at creating a mutual, genetic child with their husbands, but some women feel it is unfair to have to do the lion's share of the work to get pregnant. Husbands, too, often feel guilty at putting their wives through IVF. Here is another place where seeing yourselves as a team may help your coping.

> Veejay was 36 years old and his wife, Sima, 31 when they found out that he had an extremely low sperm count. The couple was told that their chances of conceiving through sexual intercourse were almost nil. Their infertility program estimated their chances of bringing home a baby from a cycle of IVF-ICSI as about 1 in 3. Since Sima appeared to have normal fertility, she had a very high chance of getting pregnant if the couple chose donor insemination. Sima had never had a major illness or surgery, but her mother had died of cancer when Sima was 10, leaving the little girl with an intense fear of doctors and hospitals. Sima wanted a child very badly, and had gritted her teeth and tolerated the medical tests she had to endure for the infertility workup. The thought of having a daily hormone injection and repeated ultrasound tests and pelvic examinations was unbearable to her, however. She begged Veejay to agree to donor insemination. She reminded him that a son might inherit Veejay's infertility, since it was possible that his low sperm count was genetic. She told him that being a father was 99 percent raising a child and only 1 percent providing the sperm cell. She pointed out that if they did not have to spend $8,000 for an IVF cycle, they would have enough savings for a down payment on a house, one of the goals they had wished to achieve before becoming parents.
>
> Veejay was not convinced, however. He worried that he would be unable to truly love a child who was not genetically his, but would always be looking for the sperm donor's looks and personality traits. Since Veejay's family were very conscious of issues relating to culture and religion, he knew they would not accept a child born of donor insemination, yet he also could not imagine deceiving his parents and sisters about the child's background, whereas Sima felt that privacy about donor insemination was the best option.
>
> Neither Sima nor Veejay was ready to consider living without a child, and neither was very enthusiastic about adoption, partly

because it was not well accepted in their ethnic community. Whenever they tried to talk about choosing between IVF-ICSI and donor insemination, however, the conversation ended with Sima crying and Veejay retreating to his computer.

The couple told their infertility specialist about their dilemma and were referred to a psychologist familiar with the infertility program. He helped the partners find some common ground. Veejay had not realized how scared Sima felt about the medical aspects of IVF. The psychologist offered to teach her relaxation techniques to help manage her anxiety at the hospital, and Veejay volunteered to give her injections, which was less anxiety-provoking to Sima than injecting herself. The IVF program had begun to use a progesterone vaginal gel, which eliminated the painful progesterone-in-oil shots that she had been dreading. Sima agreed to try one cycle of IVF, and Veejay promised not to pressure her to attempt a second stimulation cycle if the first one failed. Both partners were willing to freeze any extra embryos to be used in a transfer cycle.

Veejay, in turn, agreed to try donor insemination if the IVF attempt was not successful. His decision was helped when the psychologist gave the couple a book to read about donor insemination. Veejay was reassured that a father could love and value children that were not his own genetically. The couple did have a successful pregnancy after their first frozen embryo transfer cycle, however, so Veejay did not need to test his feelings.

DEALING WITH YOUR INFERTILITY
SPECIALISTS AS A TEAM

In this section, we focus on how you can present yourselves as a team in dealing with medical specialists. What if one or both of you begin to doubt your doctors' judgment? What if your doctor does not return your phone calls or answer your questions to your satisfaction? What if you are considering getting a second opinion or switching your care to another clinic? Some general suggestions follow.

- As often as possible, both partners should be present for medical visits, especially for discussions about treatment options. Not only does such mutuality create team spirit for solving the infertility problem, but then you will both hear what the doctors have to say, and can help each other make sure you understand their advice.

- Do not ask your doctors to keep secrets from your spouse. Maybe you think your husband's ego or your wife's self-esteem is too fragile to bear the harsh reality of the diagnosis, but you cannot protect your spouse by asking your physician to fudge the truth. You can instead be supportive about your spouse's emotional reactions.

- If your spouse's behavior concerns you—for example, if you worry that your spouse is getting deeply depressed or is not following medical instructions accurately—talk to your spouse before you alert your medical team. Whenever possible, it is best to make an appointment so you and your spouse can discuss these issues jointly with your physician.

- If you believe your physicians, the nurses, or other members of the infertility team are not communicating clearly, discuss with your spouse how the two of you can be assertive in getting your needs met. Again, scheduling a joint, face-to-face visit to get answers for your concerns is best. You can help each other to avoid passive acceptance of inadequate communication, as well as managing to express your feelings clearly, without getting belligerent or tearful.

- If you are thinking of making a change to a different clinic, try to agree as much as possible between yourselves on your strategy before you present it to your doctors. You do not want to come across as a couple in which the "good spouse" likes the care you are getting, but the "bad spouse" wants to change because of perfectionism or unrealistic expectations. Remember that your medical records belong to you. A clinic or a physician should always agree to your requests to see your records or have them sent to another medical facility.

DEALING WITH INSENSITIVE
FAMILY MEMBERS AND FRIENDS

One of the most painful aspects of infertility is the need to cope with insensitive or occasionally downright hostile remarks by people who should be on your side.

Although there are many ways to cope with such people, it is crucial to try to do so as a team. Usually the people most likely to come between spouses are the in-laws. Chances are that you feel angry and frustrated if your husband's mother is making snide remarks about your choosing

THE INFERTILITY PATIENT'S
"10 MOST UNWANTED LIST"

- Parents who ask you when they can expect to have a grandchild
- Pregnant women who complain about their pregnancy symptoms
- Parents of small children who complain about their stress and sleep deprivation
- Men who boast about their sperm count or fertility
- People who say you must be enjoying your childfree lifestyle and having all that extra money
- People who tell you to accept that infertility must be God's plan for you
- People who tell you to just relax or go on a vacation and you will get pregnant
- People who give you media articles about negative aspects of infertility treatment
- People who create unwanted pregnancies
- Anyone who abuses or even browbeats a child

to work full-time instead of having a baby, and the reality is that you have been trying to conceive for three years; your husband has no sperm in his semen; and he is adamant that his family not be told. At least he could agree to tell his mother assertively that you and he have made joint decisions about having children, and that she must stop making remarks that hurt your feelings. Remember that when it comes to dealing with annoying family or friends, in a healthy marriage the first priority should be your spouse's feelings.

Another principle is to be assertive with people. Occasionally, if an insensitive remark comes from a casual acquaintance or a coworker, the path of least resistance is just to ignore it. But with people whom you see often, or who repeatedly say or do things to make you feel worse about your fertility, you need to tackle the communication calmly and directly.

Example 1.   Bill's father, a strongly religious man, tells him for the third time: "I just know that the Lord would give you a child if you went to church and prayed regularly. If you hadn't married a Catholic, I'm sure you'd go more often like you used to."

An assertive response would be: "Dad, I know you are trying to express your concern for Irene and me, but that kind of remark just makes me feel worse. I will go to church when it feels right to me. I also don't like it when you blame Irene for my choices about religion. If you feel prayers would be helpful, then I hope you will pray for us."

Example 2.   Matilda's fellow teachers all sit around in the lounge at lunch and complain about how much they are spending on clothes for their children. One of the other women says to Matilda, "Hey that's a really nice dress you're wearing. I guess it must be nice to be able to spend your money on yourself."

Matilda does not want to discuss her attempts to have a child with her coworkers, but she replies, "You're assuming I have no children because I would rather spend money on myself. Imagine how I might feel if I couldn't have a baby and you made that remark to me?"

Coworker: "Oh, I'm sorry. I guess I didn't think. Are you having a problem?"

Matilda: "I think that choices about having children are very private, and I don't feel like discussing mine."

This chapter looked at the interpersonal side of infertility. The focus was on communication and feelings within yourself or between partners. After fighting the battle of infertility, however, a couple may find that their enjoyment of sex has become a casualty. The next chapter suggests some ways to heal your sex life, with or without a baby on board.

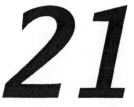

Healing Your Sex Life after Male Infertility

Infertility typically does not enhance a couple's sex life. In fact, the stress of having intercourse on demand at midcycle, the stress and invasion of privacy in undergoing repeated genital examinations and other medical tests, and sadness that natural sexual intercourse is unlikely to result in pregnancy often reduce one or both partners' interest in sex. This chapter offers some ways to repair damage to your sex life during infertility treatment, so that temporary problems do not become permanent.

SEX: MORE THAN
A MEANS TO CONCEPTION

Sex can serve many purposes. Obviously, human sexual behavior evolved to carry on our species by producing pregnancy. If you look at the animal world, however, you see that in higher animals, such as the primates, sexual interactions also strengthen social ties, cement the power hierarchy within a group, reduce anxiety and aggression, and include sexual acts that appear to occur for pleasure at nonfertile times. Humans, the most sophisticated of the primates, have the most complicated sex lives. Our use of language allows sex to have symbolic meaning beyond the sheer physical experience.

When couples are undergoing infertility diagnosis and treatment, they tend to zero in on having sex to achieve pregnancy. Often, the time and effort you put into foreplay decreases. You end up having quickies at midcycle, and periods of no sex in between. Instead of being prompted to get some lovemaking going because of sexual desire, you initiate it because it is the right day of the month or the ovulation stick turned blue.

FROM LUSTY TO LISTLESS

When you are trying to have sex on demand to conceive, you may find that lovemaking no longer makes the two of you feel more intimate and close. It may not even be very much fun. It is serious business, the X on the calendar chart you will have to show to your doctor (and many couples pencil in a few extra Xs if the monthly calendar looks too empty), not a time for giggling or back rubs. Instead of looking into each other's eyes, you are looking at the clock, thinking, "Let's get this over with so I can get some sleep."

If you ever longed for marriage to put an end to guilt over sex without a religious and legal sanction, or anticipated the day you could throw away the pills, condoms, diaphragms, and gels, you probably never imagined sex could become such a chore.

Then there are the mental images that infertility brings. To enjoy sex, you need to be able to concentrate on its pleasures. In the middle of trying to focus on your bodily tingles or your attraction to your partner (or even on a sexual fantasy that would normally really turn you on), comes the picture of your sperm cells as a bunch of dead and dying tadpoles, or your cervical mucus as a thicket as hostile and full of thorns as the one around Sleeping Beauty's castle. You see in your mind's eye the rosy newborn in the hospital nursery that will never be yours or you think about your sister-in-law's pregnant belly.

MALE PERFORMANCE PROBLEMS

It is not surprising, especially when infertility has gone on for months or years, that men sometimes develop difficulty maintaining erections or reaching orgasm at the most crucial times of the month. Typically, everything goes smoothly if a couple tries sex during a week when conception is unlikely. When the calendar, the thermometer, or the ovulation kit says "now is the time," however, sex becomes a command performance. Sometimes the crucial days are busy ones, and the only time to have sex is very early in the morning, or late at night when the couple is exhausted. Even if their schedule is lighter, planning sex can take away the sense of spontaneity and arousal.

For men, having anxious thoughts about erections can almost instantaneously create an erection problem. Negative thoughts about being unable to get or keep an erection generate negative feelings, such as anxiety and shame. The feelings lead to more negative thoughts. The brain sends a message to the penis: "Hey! Something is wrong! Forget about sex and get ready to fight or run!" The erection does a disappearing act. Some men experience lifelong erection problems. They need medical or psychological treatment. For most, however, this is just a temporary difficulty that occurs in reaction to various pressures, such as trying for a pregnancy.

Some men have a slightly different problem. They can stay relaxed enough to keep a firm erection, but cannot manage to ejaculate during intercourse, even if they keep thrusting for 30 or 45 minutes. Often ejaculation is just fine during a man's own private masturbation.

LOSS OF PLEASURE FOR WOMEN

Infertility also can create sexual problems for women, but unless a loss of desire interferes with having intercourse at the right time, a woman's sexual function usually does not limit her chance of becoming pregnant. A woman can have intercourse without being mentally aroused at all. The most common problem women experience physically during infertility is lack of vaginal lubrication. Normally, using a water-based vaginal lubricant makes intercourse quite comfortable, but when a couple is trying to conceive, *lubricants must be avoided because they slow down or kill sperm cells.* Spending a longer time on foreplay, or thinking erotic thoughts, can often improve a woman's arousal and lubrication, however.

As we discussed in chapter 6, there is no scientific evidence that having an orgasm during intercourse improves a woman's chance of pregnancy, so the main mechanical issue is avoiding pain and irritation. Of course, it would also be very preferable if the woman enjoyed each sexual experience!

MAKING SEX SPECIAL AGAIN

For the sake of both partners, your sex life may need some tender loving care during or after infertility treatment. If you put a priority on making sex romantic, playful, and relaxed, you can often recapture the pleasure that has been missing and reverse the problems that are interfering with a more satisfying sex life. Here are some suggestions.

- Make sure you have sex at times of the month besides midcycle. If you know conception is very unlikely on a certain day, go ahead and use a lubricant, have orgasms from oral sex or hand caressing, or do anything else you were omitting out of fear it would interfere with pregnancy.

- Help set the mood for sex by making the setting special, and by taking time to separate yourselves from the stress of your busy lives. For example, put scented candles in the bedroom, put on some music you both like, have sex in front of the fireplace, start by taking a shower or bubble bath together, or exchange back rubs.

- Don't be afraid to tell your partner with words or gestures how and where you would like to be touched. Take some time during lovemaking to lie back and focus on your own pleasure. At other moments you can make a special effort to excite your partner.

- You may want to tell each other your sexual fantasies, read an erotic story out loud, or watch a sexy movie together. Some couples enjoy games that are designed to enhance sex, or wearing special lingerie.

- If you have been having a problem keeping erections or reaching orgasm, give yourself a vacation from intercourse. Make an agreement at the beginning of lovemaking that penetration is not on the menu. Instead, let each partner have a turn to lie back and enjoy being caressed with no pressure to get an erection for the man, or to reach orgasm for the man or the woman. If one of you wants to have an orgasm, limit the options to hand caressing or oral sex so that having an erection is not a requirement. If this strategy helps to reduce the pressure to perform, try it several times until you both feel more relaxed and confident before going back to having intercourse.

- If a problem with erections or inability to ejaculate persists, an excellent self-help book, *The New Male Sexuality* (see "Resources"), presents some step-by-step exercises for couples that can help you get back to normal.

FINDING PROFESSIONAL HELP

If sexual problems do not clear up despite efforts to change your sexual routine, you may need to find some professional help. If you are fairly sure that the problem is based on anxiety or stress, a mental health professional trained in sex therapy can often help couples improve their sex lives, using an action-oriented, short-term type of treatment. The therapist meets with both members of the couple, giving them homework exercises to try in the privacy of their home. A trained sex therapist should be a fully credentialed mental health professional; that is, a doctoral-level, licensed psychologist, a board-certified psychiatrist, or a licensed social worker or counselor. You will often find professionals who have special training in treating sexual problems in large cities, or on the faculty of a medical school's department of psychiatry, gynecology, or urology. National organizations, such as the Society for Sex Therapy and Research (SSTAR) or the American Association of Sex Educators, Counselors, and Therapists, may also be able to refer you to members in your area (see "Resources").

If you think a medical problem, such as low hormone levels, nerve damage, or poor blood flow to the penis, is causing an erection problem, you can consult a urologist with a special interest in treating sexual dysfunction. A number of medical treatments can restore firm erections without damaging fertility, including taking a medication such as sildenafil (Viagra), injecting a medication into the soft tissue of the penis to produce an erection, or having surgery to insert an inflatable penile prosthesis.

A woman who is having pain during intercourse or a severe loss of sexual desire may want to consult her gynecologist, although again, not all gynecologists are knowledgeable about sexual problems, so you may need a referral to one who has some special training or skills in that area.

To find a urologist or a gynecologist with the interest and the skill in diagnosing and treating sexual problems, you may want to ask your family physician or your infertility specialist for a referral. Again, county medical associations or local medical schools are another referral source.

WHAT IF YOU GET PREGNANT?

When couples finally achieve a pregnancy after infertility treatment, many worry about any activity that might promote a miscarriage. One of the activities couples frequently give up is sex. In most situations, however, it is perfectly safe to stay sexually active during pregnancy. Exceptions include times when a woman is having symptoms of a threatened miscarriage, or if the sac that holds the amniotic fluid has ruptured at the very end of pregnancy (waters have broken) but labor has not yet begun, or any other time that your obstetrician says you should not have sex.

During the first *trimester* (the first 13 weeks) of pregnancy, women often feel tired out or nauseated, and desire for sex may temporarily decrease. On the other hand, many women report increased sexual desire during the second trimester. Some become more easily orgasmic than before, perhaps because tiny, new blood vessels develop in the genital area.

In the third trimester, a woman's increasing belly may make sex awkward or uncomfortable. Sometimes couples need to find new positions for intercourse or may prefer to bring each other to orgasm using hand caressing or oral sex. Although a woman may become more aware of the sensations of her uterus contracting during orgasm as her pregnancy progresses, having intercourse would very rarely bring on premature labor during a normal pregnancy.

IS THERE SEX AFTER CHILDREN?

Couples experiencing infertility rarely think about the negative aspects of being parents. One of them, however, is the impact on your sex life. Especially during the first year after a baby is born, both partners' sleep may be interrupted for nighttime feedings and diaper changes. Of course, this contributes to daytime fatigue. Even when a child sleeps through the night, one or both parents may keep one ear open during lovemaking for crying or other noises signaling a problem. It is not unusual for a small child to wander into your bedroom at just the wrong moment. Although modern studies show that witnessing parents having sex does no lasting damage to a toddler's psyche, it certainly may break the romantic mood for Mom and Dad!

Women often gain weight during pregnancy, and some experience other permanent changes (stretch marks, changes in hair texture, drooping breasts) in their body shape or appearance. After a baby is born, it may take a while to feel as attractive as before. Sometimes just becoming a parent changes a woman's or a man's self-concept about being sexy. Although breast-feeding is important to a baby's health, and may have temporary positive sexual benefits in increasing breast size or erotic sensitivity, it also can interfere with sexual pleasure. Some women have trouble switching gears from using their breasts as feeding stations to thinking of them as pleasure zones. During breast-feeding, hormonal changes include a reduced level of estrogen, often causing vaginal dryness and irritation with intercourse. Now that pregnancy has been accomplished, get out that water-based lubricant again!

So the bottom line is: If you are going through infertility, pay some attention to keeping your sex life vital. It helps maintain your sense of closeness and caring as a couple when emotional times are tough. Pleasurable sex reminds you that you did not get married only to produce children together. And you might as well put some priority on good sex while you try to get pregnant, because if you succeed, chances are that your sex life will temporarily be simmering on the back burner!

Sexuality is an area of life closely linked with values about religion and spirituality. In the next chapter, we focus on how your beliefs about spirituality and ethics may be challenged by the infertility experience.

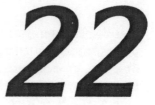

The Spiritual and Ethical Side of Infertility

Finding out that it will be difficult or even impossible to have a child forces men and women to confront their beliefs about the meaning of life. In other chapters, we detail the major religions' interpretations about masturbation to produce semen, insemination with husband's or donor's sperm, assisted reproductive technology (ART), and cryopreserving embryos. Here we want to talk about more general issues regarding making spiritual sense of infertility.

THE "WHY ME?" QUESTION

It is a rare man or woman diagnosed with infertility who has never asked, "Why me?" Surrounded by people who conceive without much thought or effort, and often are so unappreciative of their children, you may wonder whether the condition resulted from a past misdeed, bad luck, divine intention, or random fate.

Some people believe that infertility is a punishment for something in one's past. The punishment theory may appeal to you if you picture God as a supreme being intimately involved in your daily life, micromanaging the universe. Viewing infertility as a personal chastisement is not a helpful coping strategy, however, as Debbie discovered.

Debbie had her wild period in high school. She binge drank and had a number of sexual partners. Looking back on it, she realized she was probably reacting to her unhappiness at home. Her mother had remarried a man who was alcoholic and periodically violent. Debbie got pregnant at age 15 as the result of a date rape. Distraught, she told her mother, who pushed Debbie into getting an abortion as quickly as possible. Her mother seemed more concerned with keeping the pregnancy a secret from Debbie's stepfather than with her daughter's feelings.

Debbie left home at 17, and after working her way through college, met and married a loving, older man when she was 25. When Debbie failed to get pregnant, she was sure it was a punishment for her previous abortion. The infertility specialists dismissed her concerns, saying there was a motility problem on the male side, as well as some ovulation dysfunction for Debbie. Debbie could not forgive herself, however. She was too upset to try hormonal stimulation, and the couple gave up on infertility treatment.

After two years had passed, Debbie still longed for a child. She made an appointment with the rabbi at her synagogue and told him the story. He helped her to forgive herself for the past, and to see that the infertility was not a punishment. The couple tried infertility treatment again, and this time a pregnancy resulted.

You may have trouble letting go of the belief that you are being punished. If you have a strong need to control your own destiny, it may be more comforting to think that you are being punished for a sin than to feel that you have no influence over your fertility. Sometimes clergy also reinforce such ideas.

Mark grew up without much religious background. His family was officially Presbyterian, but he never went to church or Sunday school. In college he began to drink heavily and use marijuana. He dropped out of school, but straightened out his life when he and his girlfriend became evangelical Christians. They married, but were unable to conceive. Mark's doctor told him he had a large varicocele. His pastor, however, said the infertility was God's payback for Mark's past years of sinful living, especially the fact that he and his wife had been sexually active while they were dating. Mark and his wife went to a variety of revival meetings and healing services, but he did not have the varicocele surgery his doctor recommended. No pregnancy occurred.

Taking control of your infertility usually means taking an active role in getting the best medical care. Being a good or righteous person may be a reward in itself, but does not guarantee a pregnancy.

INFERTILITY AND
LOSS OF RELIGIOUS FAITH

Infertility can make people question their religious faith. If there is a just God, why does he (or she) give babies to couples who mistreat and abuse them, and deny babies to good people who would make excellent parents? Infertility often makes religious people angry at God. From a strictly secular view, infertility will quickly destroy the belief that life is fair.

If you are searching for a spiritual meaning in infertility, it is often more comforting to think of it as part of a complex plan for you or a challenge, rather than as a divine slap in the face. Some couples believe that infertility is God's way of bringing them closer emotionally, or of testing their religious faith. Some believe they have been given a mission to adopt a child who needs a home rather than to be genetic parents. For example, Jewish rabbis do not regard infertility as a punishment for sins, but note that in biblical stories, God used infertility as a means of encouraging more prayer and attention to spirituality.

CLARIFYING YOUR OWN BELIEFS

If you practice an organized religion, you may find comfort in discussing the meaning of infertility with a sympathetic and insightful member of your clergy. You also may want to read religious texts and commentaries about infertility. Some religious organizations sponsor support groups for people with infertility that focus attention on spiritual issues. Sharing your thoughts with a small group of people from your congregation who discuss religious issues may also be helpful, even if other group members have not experienced infertility.

Many people also seek some meaning in life's events but do not practice an organized religion. You may find some helpful insights in the many self-help books on coping with infertility or in support groups for infertile couples. Techniques of meditation or relaxation can also provide you with opportunities to feel spiritually refreshed.

When thinking about the meaning of infertility, here are some answers that other men and women have found helpful:

- Going through infertility challenges me to value myself for all the things I can accomplish beside being a parent.

- Going through infertility challenges me to value my marriage as a partnership based on love and understanding, through thick and thin, even if we never become parents.

- There are many ways that I can help children to have happy lives, filled with caring. These include being a genetic parent, adopting a child, or finding ways to teach and care for children not my own.

- Experiencing infertility helps me empathize with people who may have even worse unhappiness—for example those who face a life-threatening illness or a permanent disability, who face war or famine, or who lose their spouses through death or divorce.

- As we go through infertility as a couple, we have the chance to feel closer by working together to solve the problem in one way or another.

- I do not have to see my infertility as neglect or punishment by a higher power. The world is clearly full of many evils that have no purpose easily understood in human terms.

- Going through infertility challenges me to define what kind of faith I have: faith in some higher purpose in life; faith that there is a God who directs all our fates; faith in luck, or even in a random world; faith in myself and my abilities to cope with what life brings.

Infertility not only challenges our belief systems and ethical values, it also demands that we examine our financial priorities. Thus we turn from the abstract concerns of spirituality to the very concrete worries of how to pay for the treatment that may result in our longed-for child.

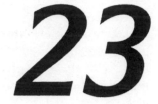

Robbing Paul to Pay Peter: The Economics of Male Infertility

In the United States, one of the most upsetting aspects of infertility is the financial strain often involved in treating it. Federal law does not require that government or private insurers pay for the costs of infertility diagnosis or treatment. At the time this book was being written, only 12 states had laws mandating some type of insurance coverage for infertility, although many private insurers offer some benefits, especially on their more expensive policies. Still, most readers who have infertility treatment will end up with large, out-of-pocket medical bills.

If you want to know the law for your state, you can contact the American Society for Reproductive Medicine (ASRM), which summarizes current state laws on its web site (see "Resources"). In general, the state laws have many loopholes, requiring coverage only by some types of insurance plans or for very limited annual medical costs. Currently, the strongest laws are in Illinois, Massachusetts, and Rhode Island.

The actual costs to insurers of paying for infertility treatment appear very reasonable. A recent analysis of insurance costs in Massachusetts showed that covering infertility accounted for less than half of 1 percent of the total health care costs in 1993 in the state's Blue Cross-

Blue Shield fee-for-service plan, despite the fact that in that year, people in Massachusetts were the most likely of any U.S. couples to use assisted reproductive technology (ART). Couples with infertility, as well as their families and friends, need to advocate for changes in the insurance laws that recognize the importance of infertility treatment. Resolve has played an important role in various states in organizing legislative campaigns across the nation (see "Resources").

Of course, once you have a baby—whether you conceive in the time-honored way, get pregnant with the help of a team of infertility experts, or adopt—you will bear the costs of raising that child: anywhere from about $100,000 for the bare necessities until age 18, to $300,000 for a more deluxe upbringing, including private college. We are not sure if this helps put the costs of infertility treatment in perspective, or just increases the size of your headache!

STRATEGIES TO MAXIMIZE INSURANCE COVERAGE

Before you begin an infertility evaluation, research your insurance policy carefully to see whether it covers any services related to infertility. Read your whole insurance contract, including the fine print and the list of medical procedures that are *excluded* in your policy. If two spouses each have different insurance, consider whether to seek coverage for both husband and wife under the policy that is most favorable. If you are likely to change jobs soon, compare the coverage you have now with the policy you are likely to have in your new position. Time your infertility evaluation and treatment accordingly, if you can. If you have already paid your yearly deductible amount, it may also be to your advantage to have an expensive surgery or ART procedure within that same year.

Remember that once you have a diagnosis of infertility in your medical records, it may become a preexisting condition that is not covered for some period of time if you switch to a new insurance policy. If your infertility was caused by a past medical illness—for example, by cancer chemotherapy—it may be considered a preexisting condition even if you never sought treatment for it before. Pregnancy may also be treated as a preexisting condition if you switch insurance after conceiving a baby. New federal laws guaranteeing that you can carry insurance coverage from one job to another may not help, especially since those laws do not apply to companies that insure themselves.

Some policies cover infertility diagnosis, but not treatment, or infertility treatments, but not in vitro fertilization (IVF) or other assisted reproductive technologies. Even if your insurance plan does not cover any diagnostic tests or treatments related to infertility, you may be able to get coverage for surgical procedures, laboratory tests, ultrasound examinations, or medications if your infertility specialist can bill them one by one, using a legitimate diagnosis that may not involve infertility per se. Many infertility clinics have billing specialists who can help you get the maximum reimbursement possible.

If your insurance company denies a claim, ask them to give you information in writing about the reason for their refusal to pay. Before you begin infertility treatment, ask the clinic to submit a letter to your insurance company asking for predetermination of benefits. The letter should itemize all the procedures that will be done, the fee for each, and the medical reason for each. Sadly, if the infertility clinic you have chosen does not provide help with insurance issues, you may want to consider going elsewhere for your treatment.

One of the pharmaceutical companies that manufactures hormones for ART, Organon, offers an infertility insurance advice hot line that is free of charge to any infertility patient (see "Resources").

DO NOT DROP COVERAGE TO SAVE MONEY!

We sometimes have seen patients who are young and healthy, other than the infertility, drop their usual health insurance coverage to save money to invest in infertility treatment. This is a terrible idea. You could be injured, get an infection, or be diagnosed with an unsuspected serious illness at any time. Furthermore, you hope your infertility treatment will result in a pregnancy. If a woman becomes pregnant without having medical insurance, she usually will not be able to buy insurance after conception to cover her prenatal care and delivery. Especially given the high costs of multiple pregnancies from ART, this is the last time in your life you would want to lack insurance.

IVF PROGRAMS THAT
GUARANTEE A PREGNANCY

A few IVF programs have recently been offering a money-back guarantee. You pay a flat fee that covers a full cycle of IVF. If no pregnancy results by the end of the cycle, you get most of your money back. Such programs typically have strict criteria for accepting patients. They only offer the guarantee to couples who are likely to have a pregnancy; for example, those with a wife under age 35. The flat fee they charge is often 150 percent to 220 percent more than you would pay for a cycle at another good IVF program. They guarantee a pregnancy that will be viable through the first trimester, but do not guarantee the birth of a live baby. The refund you receive in the case of failure usually does not include the costs of diagnostic tests to evaluate you for your cycle or of the infertility medications.

The ethics committee of the American Society for Reproductive Medicine recently ruled that such programs are not unethical, since they may offer patients with no health insurance the opportunity to try IVF and still have enough money to pursue another option, such as adoption, if IVF fails. As the committee noted, however, having accurate information about the costs and benefits of these programs is crucial. Do careful comparison shopping before you invest in a guarantee. Look in detail at the conditions for getting your money back. What if the pregnancy ends in miscarriage or your baby is stillborn? Are there treatment costs, such as medication, that are not included in the flat fee? What are the success rates versus the costs of the program compared to others that do not offer a guarantee? Does the program tend to transfer more than two or three embryos, which might increase their pregnancy rates but also increases your risk of a multiple gestation with all its complications?

WHEN PARTNERS DISAGREE ABOUT
MONEY FOR INFERTILITY TREATMENT

Because most couples with infertility have to pay some or all of the cost of their treatment, it is not unusual for partners to have different ideas

about how much money to invest in expensive and uncertain procedures. In our experience, the husband more commonly rates the infertility treatment lower on his priority list than does his wife, but sometimes the disagreement goes the other way. Perhaps one partner is
frightened by the risk of taking a home equity loan or depleting retire-
ment funds in the search to have a baby. He or she is thinking of the
good of the family in the long term. This can be a particularly tough
issue if you already have one child and disagree on how much to invest
in trying to have a second.

Children are very crucial to the happiness of many couples, however. Perhaps you feel you could live more contentedly in a small apart-
ment with a child than in a lovely house with an empty crib. Or maybe
you have a tough time worrying about money in your old age when your
most important goal now is to be a parent. The two of you need to negotiate to find a level of risk you both can tolerate. Perhaps one or both
partners would be willing to take a second job for awhile to save up for
IVF or adoption, or maybe there is an ultimate dollar limit to the infertility treatment that you can both endorse. Some couples calculate the
cost of an adoption and make sure that they would have enough money
left to pursue that option after trying infertility treatment.

A more thorny problem occurs when one partner likes to have
money for luxuries, such as vacations, jewelry, or a sports car, instead of
paying for an expensive infertility procedure. The difference in your values is only likely to widen if you are successful in having a child, because
family life interferes with fun and spontaneity. Sometimes a focus on
material things is also a way of coping with grief about infertility. If you
and your partner have a fundamental difference in your priorities in life,
this is an excellent time to seek some counseling as a couple with a mental health professional who can help you understand each other and
compromise more effectively. Otherwise, this particular conflict can
break up a relationship.

INFERTILITY INVESTMENT COUNSELING

Cost-effectiveness is one of the bywords of modern medicine: not only
must treatments work, but they should be as economical as possible.
Particularly with the success of in vitro fertilization with intracytoplasmic sperm injection (IVF-ICSI), controversies about cost-effectiveness
have developed in the treatment of male infertility. Should you try some

cycles of superovulation or go right to IVF-ICSI? Should you have your vasectomy reversed surgically, or just have IVF-ICSI with sperm retrieved from your epididymis? Should varicoceles be repaired, or should you just undergo ART if you have a low sperm count and motility?

When trying to calculate the cost-effectiveness of any infertility treatment, there are many factors that come into the equation. It is not always possible to make absolute comparisons between one procedure and another, or indeed between one hospital and another. Hospital costs and fees for surgery and anesthesia vary widely across the United States. It is generally less expensive to do surgery in a special outpatient unit than in a large hospital. Today, most hospitals associated with universities and major teaching centers have built combined outpatient surgicenters, requiring less personnel and not offering the intensive monitoring that the sicker patients need. On the other hand, major medical teaching centers, and their expert staff, are located in larger cities, where the cost of living is higher, making the cost of medical care greater as well.

Superovulation versus IVF.   Studies have looked at the cost-effectiveness of several cycles of superovulation (intrauterine insemination, or IUI, with the woman taking injectable hormones) versus going right to IVF-ICSI for infertility due to a male problem. A consensus is that three cycles of superovulation (which might average about $1,000 to $1,500 a cycle) is more cost-effective before trying IVF-ICSI (which may cost around $7,000 to $10,000, including all medications, in 1999 dollars), as long as a man's semen quality meets the criteria that give superovulation a reasonable chance of success (see chapter 16). Superovulation not only may get you a baby for a cheaper average cost than IVF-ICSI, but there are fewer medical risks to the female partner. If a man's sperm motility and count are very poor, however, or there are other signs predicting fertilization failure, IVF-ICSI remains the treatment of choice.

Vasectomy Reversal versus IVF-ICSI with Epididymal Sperm.   The success of IVF-ICSI started a small battle between reproductive endocrinologists, who saw a way to treat male infertility without even involving a urologist, and the urologic surgeons, who believed it was better to present the results of each approach to patients and then to let the couple decide. Each side said their treatment was more cost-effective. Several experts have analyzed both the theoretical costs and the success rates of the two treatments and some actual outcomes in real life. Since we are from the urology camp, we are pleased to report that vasectomy reversal wins hands down, turning out to be less expensive and more effective, even if a second operation is needed because the first was unsuccessful.

There are some conditions, however, that would lead us to favor IVF-ICSI. If the vasectomy was performed more than 14 years ago, a reversal has more limited success (see chapter 10). If a vasectomy reversal succeeded, but the semen quality is not optimal or there are high levels of antisperm antibodies, IVF-ICSI may be the best option. The success of vasectomy reversal is also very dependent on the skill of the surgeon. If you do not have access to an expert microsurgeon, but are able to use a highly successful clinic that provides IVF-ICSI, take the resources available (including the insurance coverage in your individual case) into account.

A couple of years ago, physicians at Cornell University Medical Center and the Cleveland Clinic independently looked at the costs of surgery for vasectomy reversal and compared it to the then current live birth rate obtained with sperm aspiration and in vitro fertilization with ICSI. Not only was the cost of the surgery or the IVF-ICSI procedure included, but also the hospital costs for the delivery, time off from work for the parents, and most important, the cost related to caring for the infant in the hospital, a sum that can skyrocket with the multiple births that are so much more common with IVF-ICSI. The comparable cost for a live birth was $25,475 for vasectomy reversal, with 47 percent of couples having a baby within the specified time period, and $72,521 for ICSI, with a delivery rate after one cycle of 33 percent. When we looked at our patients who required the more complex and more expensive vasoepididymostomy rather than simple vasovasostomy for vasectomy reversal, the cost differential was equally striking. For the reversal surgery, the cost per live birth was $31,099. In comparison, averaging the percentage of live births from various studies as a result of sperm aspiration and IVF-ICSI, the cost was $51,024.

These costs have been averaged, and should not be confused with the actual amount an individual patient might pay for a procedure. Individual fees for each procedure are difficult to tabulate. In our experience, they vary by locale and institution or surgeon. Much of the added expense with IVF-ICSI is due to the higher rate of multiple births. As reproductive endocrinologists develop methods to improve pregnancy rates while transferring fewer embryos, the cost per live birth with IVF-ICSI should come down.

Treating Varicoceles versus IVF-ICSI.   Some infertility experts have also advocated skipping surgery or embolization for a varicocele (see chapter 12) in favor of using IVF-ICSI to bypass the problem of poor semen quality. Again, the cost-effectiveness of treating a varicocele turns out to be very much superior to simply using IVF-ICSI. Another study from the group at Cornell compared the cost per live birth of patients undergoing varicocele surgery and establishing pregnancies through intercourse versus couples who chose IVF-ICSI. With varicocele repair, the cost per live birth was $26,268 compared to $89,091 with ICSI.

Remember, too, that you may want more than one child. If repairing a varicocele results in a permanent improvement in semen quality, your family building can proceed. If you depend on IVF-ICSI, you may have to pay for a new cycle to have another child, unless you have extra cryopreserved embryos to use in trying to conceive again.

MONEY CAN BUY YOUR GENES

This chapter looked at cost-effectiveness issues comparing various medical treatments for infertility. Couples also balance issues of cost against their wish to have their own genetic offspring. IVF-ICSI is expensive and medically complex, but offers the chance for two partners to combine their genes in creating a child. Some see this opportunity as priceless. Others choose donor insemination because it is inexpensive and entails few risks for the woman in the couple. Making such choices means juggling your financial resources and your personal beliefs about nature and nurture in parenting.

Another alternative is to adopt a genetically unrelated child. Adoption is highly valued in our society because we see it as giving love and opportunity to a child who might otherwise be unwanted or neglected. Adoption has also become increasingly expensive and complex, however, as we see in the next chapter.

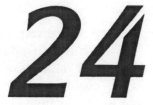

Choosing to Adopt a Child

Adoption in one form or another is probably as old as human history. In our child-centered society, adoption unites a child who needs a family with parents who want a child to nurture and love. According to Adoptive Families of America, 2.2 percent of families in the United States, or 1.5 million families, have adopted a child. Each year, 50,000 to 60,000 children are adopted by families not related to them. About half of these children are adopted in infancy.

ADOPTION THROUGH AN AGENCY

The most common way to adopt is through a public or private adoption agency. The agency has social workers and other trained professionals who evaluate the couple wishing to adopt, counsel the birth parents, and make sure all relevant state, federal, or international laws are followed. Each agency has its own criteria for choosing among the many families who want to adopt a child. Most will not give a couple a child more than 40 years younger than the oldest of the prospective parents. This means that a couple in which one spouse is over age 40 may not be able to adopt an infant from many agencies.

Agencies tend to specialize in certain types of children. Some help couples adopt children from foreign countries. Others only do domestic adoptions or place mostly children with special needs (i.e., school-age children, children with disabilities or chronic illnesses, siblings who need to be adopted into one family, or children with a history of neglect or abuse). Some are affiliated with a particular religious organization and may (or may not) favor parents of that denomination. Agencies differ in whether they prefer *closed adoptions,* in which there is no contact between birth parents and adoptive parents, or *open adoptions,* in which birth parents and adoptive parents communicate, often meeting in person.

Although most adoption agencies are honest, scandals and rip-offs do occur. Adoption organizations advise couples to check the department in the agency's state that licenses adoption agencies and the state's department of social services to see how many complaints have been received about an agency. Find out how many children are placed each year by the agency and compare the fees different agencies charge. A list of state adoption units is available through the Adoptive Families of America (see "Resources"). Local adoption support groups can also give you information about the agencies serving your community. If you work with an adoption agency in a different state, make sure you research adoption laws in both your home state and the agency state.

INDEPENDENT ADOPTIONS

About half of infant adoptions are *independent*—that is, adoptive parents use an attorney or other adoption professional to find a child outside of the agency system. Many attorneys specializing in adoption belong to the American Academy of Adoption Attorneys (see "Resources"). An attorney is very important in making sure that all state laws are followed during the adoption process. In some independent adoptions, birth parents and adoptive parents connect through advertisements in newspapers or the Internet and then find an attorney to help them complete the adoption. Agencies can also help the two sets of parents with the rest of the adoption process. This is often called *directed adoption.*

In an independent adoption, the parties involved may not necessarily be required to have a home study (an interview and a home visit by a social worker to evaluate the adoptive parents) or any other type of pre-adoption counseling. While this may seem like a relief or an opportunity to save money, it also may leave birth or adoptive parents unprepared for the emotions they will experience as adoption proceeds. Many states allow potential adoptive parents to pay the medical bills and/or living expenses of the birth mother during her pregnancy when a directed adoption is planned. If she then decides to keep her baby, the money often cannot be reclaimed. Information from an insurance agency that sells policies to reimburse couples for these losses suggests that about 20 percent of these agreements fall through in the end.

Usually it is the birth mother who changes her mind, but several high-profile court cases in recent years occurred when a birth father claimed he was not given a chance to assert his parental rights. Many states now have *putative father registries* so that a man who thinks he fathered a child can register his interest in the child and be informed of any legal action concerning that child. With modern techniques of genetic testing, paternity can be legally proved. Some adopting parents may ask that the birth father named by the birth mother take a paternity test to ensure that when he gives up his parental rights, the adoption is free and clear. Otherwise, there remains a possibility that another man could claim to be the father and try to gain custody of the child. Once an adoption is finalized by the court, however, less than 1 percent are contested.

Having an experienced mental health professional meet with the birth mother or the birth parents is very helpful in making an independent adoption go smoothly. Adoptive parents should also make sure they have a chance to talk to knowledgeable professionals about their expectations and feelings.

INTERNATIONAL ADOPTIONS

In 1997, couples in the United States adopted 13,620 children from overseas. The State Department will only allow the adoption of children under age 15. The child must either have been abandoned, have only one living parent who gives the child up, or be an orphan. The two most common sources of children in 1997 were Russia and China, with South Korea third. About 60 percent of international adoptions involve a baby less than a year old, and another 30 percent are children one to four years old. Couples with infertility often consider international adoption because they are frightened by the idea that a domestic adoption might fall through or be contested. Those who prefer a closed adoption are relieved to think that birth parents are very unlikely to search for their child in the future or intrude on the adoptive family's privacy.

In some countries, such as China, infants available for adoption are typically healthy, but have been abandoned because daughters are considered less desirable than sons, and governmental policies only allow families to raise one child. In Russia, infants are only available for international adoption if they have some type of health problem. In some eastern European or Latin American countries, children available for adoption may have experienced both physical and emotional deprivation. Sometimes this just leaves a child with delays in the development of speech or motor skills, but some children's ability to attach emotionally to adoptive parents may have been damaged. Some medical schools now offer special international adoption clinics that help families evaluate the health information they receive about children available for adoption and also provide pediatric and mental health services for the children once they arrive.

COSTS OF ADOPTING

The financial cost of adopting a child is extremely variable. Public agency adoptions may only cost several thousand dollars. When a couple adopts a child with special needs, state or federal subsidies may even be available. In 1992, however, the average cost of a domestic infant adoption in the United States was $9,200. Costs of independent adoption are typically higher, because they include attorney's or broker's fees, costs for counseling or home studies that a state may require, and—in some states—paying the birth mother's medical or living expenses. International adoptions can cost up to $35,000. Some countries require that the adoptive parents come in person to claim the child and spend a certain amount of time there before bringing the child home.

TRENDS IN THE AVAILABILITY
OF CHILDREN FOR ADOPTION

In the year 1996, a total of 3,891,494 births were recorded in the United States. About a third of these, or 1,260,306, were babies born to unmarried women. Estimates are that another 1,400,000 women choose abortion to end an unwanted pregnancy each year in the United States. Of the pregnancies carried to term, perhaps 10 percent are unwanted, but far fewer than 120,000 babies are given up for unrelated adoption. In fact, if about 200,000 couples seek to adopt an unrelated infant each year, only about 1 in 7 will succeed.

The number of healthy babies available for domestic U.S. adoption will probably continue to decrease. The rates of births to young, unmarried women are falling every year. Surveys from the 1980s showed that unmarried and pregnant Caucasian women who gave up babies for adoption were less likely to have been in the workforce, were more likely to be students, were somewhat older than other pregnant girls, and had mothers with higher educational levels—traits suggesting a higher social status that might be desirable to adopting parents. These women were more likely to give up daughters than sons. We do not have more recent surveys to compare to these statistics, which are now over 10 years old. The number of international adoptions continues to climb each year, however.

TRANSRACIAL ADOPTION

Studies of minority children adopted into Caucasian families suggest they have very good overall emotional adjustment, ethnic sense of identity, and academic performance. Laws appear to be changing in the direction of allowing more transracial adoptions to take place. Many minority adoption professionals still oppose transracial adoption, however, feeling that the ideal is to match the ethnicity of child and parents. African American or Hispanic families may be unjustly excluded from adopting available children if they do not meet home study criteria because of their economic status or cultural differences from the professionals who evaluate the families. Many minority children available for adoption are older, or have been in the foster care system, rather than being given up for adoption at birth.

SPECIAL NEEDS ADOPTION

There may be as many as 100,000 children in the foster care system nationwide who are available for adoption. Most of these children fall into the special needs category. For couples who feel they have the emotional and financial resources to parent a child who may need extra reserves of acceptance, attention, patience, tutoring, or other health services, these adoptions can be extremely rewarding. Perhaps 15 percent of special needs adoptions fail, often because families feel they were not adequately prepared for the challenges that they faced. Having counseling and as much knowledge as possible about the child are crucial in making decisions about special needs adoption.

KNOWING WHAT KIND
OF ADOPTION IS RIGHT FOR YOU

Overall, the many organizations and self-help books that promote adoption present an optimistic message to potential adoptive parents: if you are willing to invest your time, money, and emotions in finding a child to adopt, you will probably succeed. Before you begin, however, you need to think about the kind of child you can nurture. How much does it matter to you to start out with an infant? To have a child of your own ethnic background? To have a child without known disabilities? To have a child who received good prenatal and postnatal care?

Attend support and networking groups in your local community for couples considering adoption. Talk to friends and acquaintances who have adopted a child. Use the Internet or order information by mail from organizations that help adoptive parents (see "Resources"). Go to the library or a bookstore and look over the many books on adoption. Most of all, talk openly to each other about your hopes and concerns about this option for having a child.

CONFRONTING YOUR FEARS
ABOUT BIRTH PARENTS

After spending months or years going through infertility treatments that violate physical and emotional privacy, many couples dread the intrusiveness of the adoption process, including having a home study, entering a mandated counseling situation, and having to impress social workers or birth parents. Even once a placement is made and the adoption is finalized legally, the adoptive parents may worry that the birth parents will keep contact with their child, perhaps interfering with parenting or somehow weakening the bond between the child and the adoptive parents.

Advocates of open adoption believe these fears are needless. Just as it is rare for the birth parents to contest a finalized adoption, it is also rare that they try to intrude in a negative fashion on the adoptive family. Having contact with the adoptive parents may reassure the birth parents that their child will have a happy life, reducing the pain of giving up the baby. One study also found that adoptive mothers who had contact with the birth mother before the baby was born had more positive attitudes both to the birth mother and to the child they adopted. Adoptive mothers who had contact with the birth mother either before the birth or in the next two years also had more positive attitudes about parenting. It is impossible to know whether these advantages stemmed from the contacts themselves, or perhaps from a trend that couples who prefer open adoption are more comfortable with the whole adoption process.

Publicity about adoptees and birth parents searching for each other also scares potential adoptive parents. It is very difficult to know how many adults who were adopted as children try to find their birth parents, but one estimate is that only about 10 percent to 15 percent do so. More women than men initiate searches, especially women who were adopted as infants. The outcome of searches varies from heartwarming stories in which the adoptee finally feels complete as a person and forges new relationships with genetic relatives to sad stories of angry parents who had no wish for contact, or who inform an adoptee that he or she was the product of rape or incest.

One survey of reunions between 114 adoptees and birth parents found that most felt the experience improved both their self-esteem and their relationship with their adoptive parents. Of course, people who respond to such a survey may be a special group. Overall, the quality of the relationship between an adopted child and the parents who raise her or him depends most strongly on the love and energy the parents invest. Some factors related to biology or to early experiences may make an adopted child more difficult to raise—but you could make the same statement about the potential for your own biological child to have emotional or physical problems.

Just as couples often consider adoption when they have exhausted other possibilities to conceive through medical treatment, they may feel ready after months or years of unsuccessful infertility therapy to rethink their need to be parents entirely. The next chapter focuses on how couples decide to live without children.

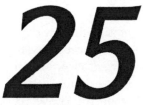

Living without Children

Although accepting a life without children is the worst fate many infertile men or women can imagine, in fact it is the future that demands the least adjustment. After all, many couples with infertility have been living without children for all the years of their relationship.

A very interesting study compared the emotions of 174 couples with infertility who succeeded in having a child with 74 couples who had children without ever having experienced infertility. The women in the infertile couples felt their overall sense of well-being had increased, but their satisfaction with their marriages actually lessened. Men in the couples with infertility also felt less satisfied with their marriages once they became parents, and did not share their wives' perception that parenthood increased their general quality of life. Compared with the couples who had experienced infertility, the "normal fertility" couples noticed fewer positive or negative changes in their life upon having a child. Perhaps the high expectations that infertile couples have about parenthood can intensify the stresses of actually having a child, as well as the joys.

THE MINUSES OF PARENTHOOD

Couples with infertility have often thought about some of the disadvantages of parenthood. Once a child is born, husbands and wives have less private time with each other. Life gets much more expensive, with money needed to feed another mouth, buy diapers and clothes, or pay a baby-sitter or school fees. Vacations and other leisure activities may no longer be affordable. Couples with children under the age of five tend to report the lowest satisfaction with their sex lives of any married group.

Sometimes husbands and wives disagree on parenting strategies. The child may seem to gravitate more to one parent or the other, or takes after your least favorite sibling. Parenting is not all kisses and carousel rides. It is also cleaning up a child who has diarrhea in the middle of the night, visits to emergency rooms for stitches, having your precious darling throw a huge tantrum in the middle of the grocery store while all the other customers watch, shelling out $30 for a tiny and undistinguished stuffed animal that took 50 cents to manufacture in Asia but has become a rare collector's item among seven-year-olds, and finding out that despite your own vows as a teenager to remain forever young and tolerant, you cannot stand the music your high schooler adores.

Although our society glorifies being a parent, not every man or woman has a mission to be a mom or dad at any cost.

FINDING THE SILVER LINING IN A CHILDFREE LIFE

If you are thinking of giving up the quest to have a child, allow yourself to think of some advantages to a life without being a parent. You will have more time, energy, and money to devote to other things that matter—including your career, hobbies, or social causes. If you want the experience of nurturing children, you can choose a profession such as teaching, nursing, or medicine that involves caring for them. You can also spend some of your free time volunteering with children who need the caring attention of an adult as a coach, tutor, big brother, or mentor. You could potentially have a significant impact on more children in your life through work or volunteering than you could as a parent.

Men or women often express fears of a lonely old age or a solitary death if they do not ever have children. In many families, however, adult children neglect their parents because the emotional bonds are not strong or geographic distance interferes. Older men and women who have warm and caring relationships with people their own age as well as younger family members, neighbors, or friends are likely to remain satisfied with their emotional contacts at the end of life.

FEELING FINISHED
WITH INFERTILITY

Many self-help books for couples with infertility point out that a grieving process occurs over time. Each treatment that fails brings you closer to the end of the line and diminishes your optimism that you will have a pregnancy. Unlike a couple whose child dies, however, or who experience a stillbirth or even miscarriage, the couple with infertility who decide to give up trying have no rituals to mark their grieving or solicit comfort from friends and family. Sometimes it may help a couple to work with a therapist or clergy person to create a prayer, meditation, or memorial service to mark the end of infertility treatment. It is also helpful to allow yourself to revel in your new freedom from doctor's visits, painful tests, having sex by the calendar, and dehumanizing exams.

REMINDING YOURSELVES OF
THE VALUE OF YOUR RELATIONSHIP

Being parents together may have been a goal you had when you made a commitment to spend your lives together. If you decide to live without children, it is important to remind yourselves of all the other needs your marriage meets. Hopefully you are each other's friend and confidant, leisure companion, chief supporter, and lover. Can you think of some other roles you fill for each other?

Whether it was only the husband who had a known fertility problem, or if you both had identified reasons why a pregnancy was not successful, the infertility affected both of your dreams and you handled it together. That is an achievement.

WHAT IF YOUR MARRIAGE BREAKS UP?

Since half of all American marriages end in divorce, some marriages split up after partners have struggled with infertility. Sometimes one partner abandons the other to start a pregnancy with someone new. Sometimes the pain of infertility is too much of a load on a fragile relationship. Probably most often, the infertility played only a minor role in the breakup of a marriage.

If you are facing the end of a marriage at the same time that you are deciding to live without children, you may experience a range of emotions, from grief to relief. It could be a good time to have some professional counseling to make sure you make good choices in the future. You may think, especially if you are a man who discovered your infertility after you married, that no other woman will ever want to marry you. In fact, dealing with infertility may be much easier when it is a fact of life discussed between dating partners before they make a commitment. In a deepening relationship, knowing about infertility can stimulate discussions of whether to seek treatment, live without children, or adopt. The answers with a new partner may be very different than the ones you found in your marriage.

BEING A STEPPARENT WHEN YOU GIVE UP THE DREAM OF A BIOLOGICAL CHILD

In this society of blended families, it is not unusual for a man or a woman to find that they are raising stepchildren, or interacting with adult stepchildren, at the same time that they are losing their dream of becoming biological parents themselves. This can happen when the husband had a vasectomy after his first marriage, or if a man with infertility marries a woman who already had children. Being a stepparent, especially when children spend a good deal of time in your household, is a challenge. You may feel your stepchildren are spoiled by your spouse or by your spouse's ex. You may resent the financial outlay spent on stepchildren. Your stepchildren may resent you and spend a good deal of energy and creativity to make your life miserable. All the normal trials of being a stepparent can be magnified when you are grieving for the loss of your own chance to have a child. If you find yourself in this type of situation, counseling as an individual or couple can often be helpful in resolving your anger.

On the other hand, a good relationship with stepchildren can help ease the grief of infertility. In the best of situations, it is similar to being an adoptive parent, especially if your spouse's ex is not a big part of the picture. When stepchildren are adults, you may at least have the chance to be a doting grandparent to their offspring.

Johanna was 37 when she married Oliver. He was 50 and had three adult sons from his first marriage. Oliver was willing to have a vasectomy reversal, but it was unsuccessful. By the time the couple exhausted lesser infertility treatments and proceeded to in vitro fertilization with intracytoplasmic sperm injection, Johanna was 40. She did not respond well to the ovarian-stimulating drugs, and no pregnancy resulted. Johanna had an active career as a violinist and felt ready to give up on further attempts at fertility treatment. She and Oliver did not feel motivated to try adoption or egg donation. At around this time, Oliver's first granddaughter was born. This son and his wife lived in the same town as Johanna and Oliver, and Johanna had become especially close to her stepdaughter-in-law. Although at first she felt tearful on holding the baby, her pleasure in being a "grandma" outweighed the pain and helped her get over the sadness of missing out on parenthood.

And now we are coming close to the end of our book. In the last chapter, we have some final thoughts about the emotional recovery from infertility.

26

Concluding Thoughts

Infertility is not just a physical state, but also a state of mind. Whether you resolve your infertility by having one or more children, by adopting, or by deciding to live without children, you need to have closure on the experience. If you are just starting out on your infertility journey, you may wonder how you could ever feel finished with it—whether you will ever be able to describe yourself without using the word "infertile."

We believe that getting closure on infertility is very important. It may involve taking some or all of the following steps:

- Do all that you can to get expert medical help from physicians you trust.

- Make resolving infertility a high priority in your life while you are actively pursuing treatment.

- Go through all the steps in infertility treatment that you and your partner mutually believe are likely to work, and that are within your sphere of personal beliefs and financial means.

- If you still have not had a child, it may be time to let go of the hope that a miracle is around the corner.

- With your life partner, weigh the pros and cons of donor insemination, adoption, and living without children. Try to make a decision that will leave you both feeling satisfied. If you cannot agree on a path, get some counseling.

- If you are not sure you are ready to stop infertility treatment, but you feel like you have hit a wall, take a break for a few months and put your priorities on another important area of your life.

- When you have made a choice, try to let go of what might have been. Celebrate your strengths and dedicate yourself to your goals, as an individual and as a couple or a family.

Although a book like this one can gather information on treating male infertility and summarize it for you, it cannot cover all the topics you might find of special interest. In addition, new advances in medicine are always taking place. The resources section that follows the glossary should give you a start on finding out extra information and updating the facts you read about in these pages.

Glossary

acromegaly An abnormal condition in which the pituitary gland makes too much human growth hormone, causing enlargement of parts of the skeleton.

acrosomal cap A caplike structure at the head of a sperm cell containing chemicals needed to penetrate into the oocyte.

acrosome reaction assay A laboratory test that measures the percentage of sperm that releases the chemicals from the acrosomal cap that aid in shell penetration.

advance directive A legal document specifying what you would want done in your medical care if you were too ill to give instructions, or what you want done with body tissues, including sperm, after your death.

alkylating drugs The category of cancer chemotherapy drugs most likely to damage male fertility, including cyclophosphamide, chlorambucil, busulfan, procarbazine, nitrosoureas, nitrogen mustard, and l-phenylalanine mustard.

amniocentesis A procedure in which an ultrasound image is used to guide a needle through the mother's uterine wall to sample the amniotic fluid that surrounds the fetus. The amniotic fluid contains living cells shed by the fetus. These cells are grown in culture and then used for genetic testing.

anabolic steroids Hormones similar to testosterone that help the human body to build up muscle mass, often illegally used to enhance athletic performance, especially strength or speed.

andrologist A specialist in studying men's sexual and reproductive function.

anejaculation Complete failure of the prostate or the seminal vesicles to squeeze out the semen and deposit it in the urethra during emission.

antioxidant therapy Using vitamins such as E, A, and C to reduce reactive oxygen species, perhaps improving semen quality.

antisperm antibodies   Chemicals made by a man's own immune system, or that of his partner, that stick to the surface of his sperm cells and damage their ability to swim or to fertilize an egg.

assisted hatching   A technique used with IVF. After embryos form, the embryologist creates a tiny opening in the outer layer of cells. Assisted hatching is believed to help the embryo to implant in the uterine lining, particularly when the woman in the couple is in her late 30s or early 40s.

assisted reproductive technology (ART)   The use of medical procedures to help conception take place outside the process of sexual intercourse.

asthenozoospermic   Having low sperm motility.

autonomic dysreflexia   A potentially life-threatening medical crisis in men with injuries high in the spinal cord, involving severe headaches, high blood pressure, and sweating, which can be brought on by an intense stimulus such as an overly full bladder, vibrator stimulation to ejaculation, or electroejaculation.

autosomal dominant   Describes a genetic syndrome in which only one parent needs to contribute a mutated gene (not on the X or Y chromosome) for offspring to have the associated disorder.

autosomal recessive   Describes a genetic syndrome in which both parents need to contribute a mutated gene (not on the X or Y chromosome) for offspring to have the associated disorder.

azoospermic   Having no sperm cells present in the semen.

balanced translocation   The transfer of a portion of one chromosome to another. Because the person with a balanced translocation has the correct amount of genetic material, he or she will not show physical abnormalities, but offspring may inherit too much or too little genetic material.

blastocyst   The stage in the growth of the embryo at about day 5 to day 7, when the cells begin to form a tiny ball.

bovine mucus penetration assay   A test using cow mucus to see whether human sperm cells can swim through it, determining the degree of sperm motility.

bulbourethral glands   Glands that produce a few drops of fluid that lubricate and prepare the urethra for ejaculation.

capacitation   A chemical process in which sperm cells finish maturing. This process generally occurs after ejaculation as the sperm swim through the cervical mucus.

carrier   Someone who is known to have a specific genetic mutation that could affect offspring, but who does not have the disease or the abnormalities that the mutation can cause.

catheter   A small, thin tube used in medical procedures; for example, to pass through the uterine cervix, to pass into the bladder, or to pass into a blood vessel.

cavernous bodies   Spongy chambers of erectile tissue in the penis that fill with blood during erection.

centrifuge   A machine used to spin liquids in the laboratory to separate their ingredients into layers of different density; employed in sperm separation.

cervical mucus   A clear, slippery substance that coats the cervix. At ovulation, the cervical mucus thins and allows sperm cells to swim through more easily.

chemical pregnancy   A blood test for hormone levels indicating that an embryo has implanted.

chorionic villus sampling (CVS)   During the first trimester of pregnancy, a needle is passed through the mother's cervix to gather a small sample of the placental tissue, which shares the same genetic makeup as the fetus. Genetic testing can then be performed on this tissue.

chromosomes   Rodlike structures within the nucleus of a cell that contain the genetic code to build a human being. Humans have 46 chromosomes: 22 pairs of autosomes and two sex chromosomes—XY in the male or XX in the female.

closed adoption   The traditional model of adoption which keeps the identity of birth parents and adoptive parents private and allows no contact between the parties.

coagulation   The normal process by which semen partially solidifies within a few minutes after ejaculation.

collagen   A protein in connective tissue that increases in the soft tissue of the penis with aging, interfering with erections.

computerized tomographic X rays (CT scans)   A way of producing very precise X-ray images of the body using a computer.

congenital bilateral absence of the vas deferens (CBAVD)   A condition in which a man is born without the vas deferens, the tube that carries sperm cells to the ejaculatory ducts from the epididymis.

congenital chordee   A birth defect in which the penis develops a curvature with erection.

corticosteroids   A group of drugs prescribed to treat intense allergic reactions, severe inflammation, or to prevent rejection of a transplanted organ.

cost-effectiveness   The expenses related to a procedure compared to how effective that procedure is; for example, the costs versus effectiveness of vasectomy reversal.

cryopreservation   The process of freezing bodily tissues, including sperm cells or embryos, in liquid nitrogen to preserve them.

cryptorchidism   A condition in which one or both testicles fail to descend into the scrotum before or shortly after birth.

crypts   Folds on the surface of the uterine cervix that provide storage space for sperm cells after ejaculation.

cumulus cells   Cloudlike cells that surround the mature oocyte.

Cushing's syndrome   A hormone problem in which the adrenal glands produce too much of the stress hormone cortisol. Men with Cushing's syndrome often have infertility related to lowered LH or testosterone.

cystic fibrosis   An autosomal recessive genetic disorder (i.e., both parents must contribute a mutated copy of the gene) that affects digestion, the pancreas, and the lungs, causing severe and chronic illness from childhood on.

cystic fibrosis transmembrane receptor (CFTR)   A gene on chromosome number 7 that, if mutated in both parents, may produce the disease cystic fibrosis in 1 out of 4 of their offspring.

cytoplasm   The fluid that surrounds the cell's nucleus and contains many other structures necessary for the cell to function.

density gradients   Layers of fluid that gradually become more solid; used in sperm separation techniques.

deoxyribonucleic acid (DNA)   The building blocks of the genetic code.

directed adoption   An adoption in which the birth mother or the birth parents choose the adoptive parents for the child.

diverticula   Abnormal pockets in the walls of a body part, such as the urethra, the bladder, or the bowel.

dopamine   A chemical (called a neurotransmitter) in the brain which carries messages from one nerve cell to another.

Down syndrome   A genetic disorder in which a baby is born with three copies, instead of two, of chromosome 21. It is more common in children born to older mothers and causes varying degrees of developmental disability and some other physical problems.

ejaculation   The second stage of the male orgasm, when semen is propelled out of the penis.

ejaculatory inevitability   The pleasant feeling that a climax is about to happen. At that moment, the smooth muscle in the walls of the prostate gland and the seminal vesicles is contracting, preparing the fluid for ejaculation.

electroejaculation   A technique that uses an electrical stimulator placed in the anal canal to trigger ejaculation.

embryo   The developing human from the time of fertilization until about the end of the second month of pregnancy. The embryo is then termed a fetus.

emission   The first stage of the male orgasm, when the ingredients in semen are mixed together by contractions of the prostate and the seminal vesicles and the vas deferens.

epididymis   A 15-foot-long tube, coiled up at the back of each testicle, in which sperm cell maturation and storage take place.

epididymitis   A painful inflammation or infection of the epididymis.

epispadias   A defect in which the urinary opening develops on the upper side of the penis instead of at the tip. It is sometimes associated with other developmental problems in the urinary system.

eugenics   The attempt to breed human beings in an effort to achieve desirable genetic qualities.

expulsion   The second stage of ejaculation, when semen is propelled by muscle contractions through the urethra and out of the penis.

fetus   The developing human from week 9 of pregnancy until birth.

flagellum   The whiplike tail of a sperm cell.

follicle-stimulating hormone (FSH)   A hormone made by the pituitary gland that controls sperm cell production in the testicles.

forward progression   The ability of the sperm cells to swim ahead briskly.

gamete intrafallopian transfer (GIFT)   An assisted reproductive procedure in which the woman undergoes ovarian stimulation and has her ripe oocytes harvested. The eggs and sperm are then deposited into her fallopian tubes.

genetic counselor   A health professional who has special training in educating patients about genetic disorders and testing. Genetic counselors must pass an examination by the American Board of Genetics Counselors to be certified.

glans   The end, or "head," of the penis, which forms a softer cushion during intercourse.

gonadotropin-releasing hormone (GnRH)   A messenger hormone produced by the hypothalamus that partially controls the pituitary's production of hormones.

granulocyte   A special type of white blood cell that appears when inflammation or infection is present. When a semen analysis indicates an abnormal level of white blood cells, too many granulocytes have been observed.

hematospermia   Blood in the semen.

hemizona assay   A test measuring the ability of the sperm cell to bind to a human egg's zona pellucida, which has been cut in half.

Huntington's disease   An autosomal dominant genetic disorder in which the central nervous system begins to deteriorate, usually in middle age.

hyperprolactinemia   A condition in which the pituitary gland makes too much of the hormone prolactin, usually because a benign tumor has developed.

hypo-osmotic swelling test   A test to identify live sperm cells, which swell when put in a fluid less salty than their interior.

hypospadias   A birth defect in which the urinary tube opens on the underside of the baby's penis instead of at the very tip.

hypothalamic-hypogonadotropic-hypogonadism   A condition in which the hypothalamus fails to produce gonadotropin-releasing hormone (GnRH).

hypothalamus   An area deep inside the brain that produces a messenger hormone that controls sperm cell production and sexual function.

hysterosalpingogram   A test in which X-ray dye is injected into the uterus so that its interior and the fallopian tubes can be seen.

immotile cilia syndrome   A rare autosomal recessive genetic disorder associated with lack of motile sperm, sinus problems, hearing loss, and decreased sense of smell.

independent adoption   An adoption arranged outside of the adoption agency system, typically with the aid of an adoption attorney.

inguinal canal   A channel on each side of the groin. The testicles slide down the canals before birth, and into the pouch of skin called the scrotum.

intracytoplasmic sperm injection (ICSI)   A procedure in which the embryologist uses a robotic microscope to insert one sperm cell into each egg harvested during in vitro fertilization.

intrauterine insemination (IUI)   A procedure in which specially prepared sperm cells are inserted directly into a woman's uterus via a small catheter passed through her cervix.

intron 8 splice 5T variant   A variation in the cystic fibrosis transmembrane receptor (CFTR) gene that is not classified as a mutation, but does contribute to about half of cases of congenital bilateral absence of the vas deferens (CBAVD).

in vitro fertilization (IVF)   An assisted reproductive technology in which a woman is given hormones to stimulate her ovaries to ripen multiple oocytes. These are harvested in an outpatient procedure and fertilized with sperm in the laboratory. Resulting embryos are transferred back into the woman's uterus.

Kallman's syndrome   A genetic condition involving developmental abnormalities in the hypothalamus that cause male infertility because of a lack of gonadotropin-releasing hormone (GnRH) production.

karyotyping   A test in which blood cells are cultured and a picture is made of the chromosomes so that their number and shape can be checked.

Klinefelter syndrome   A genetic abnormality in which men's cells have two X chromosomes and one Y (XXY). It is associated with infertility, and sometimes with specific learning disabilities and tallness.

laparoscopy   A type of surgery in which a thin telescope is inserted into the body through a small opening just below the navel, allowing the surgeon to work inside without making a larger incision.

Leydig cells   The cells in the testicles that produce the hormone testosterone.

luteinizing hormone (LH)   A hormone produced by the pituitary that stimulates the testicles to produce testosterone.

magnetic resonance imaging (MRI)   A way of producing images of the body by measuring magnetic fields.

mannose binding assay   A laboratory test that identifies whether the sperm have enough of the chemical components needed in order to bind to the zona pellucida, making fertilization possible.

meatal stenosis   A narrowing of the tip of the urethra or urinary opening that can interfere with urination and ejaculation of semen.

meatotomy   A surgical procedure to enlarge the urinary opening when it has become narrowed.

medical geneticist   A physician who has completed a special fellowship program and is board certified in this specialty.

meiosis   The special type of cell division in which a human body cell (sperm or egg) with 46 chromosomes becomes two germ cells, with only 23 chromosomes.

microdeletion   The absence of a tiny piece of genetic material from a chromosome. Microdeletions on the Y chromosome are more common in men with infertility.

microsurgery   Techniques in which a surgeon uses an operating microscope to make very tiny incisions and repairs.

microsurgical epididymal sperm aspiration (MESA)   A microsurgery in which a small incision exposes the epididymis, allowing sperm cells and fluid to be sucked out using a very fine needle and syringe.

morphology   The actual shape and size of the sperm cells, which is reported as the percentage of sperm cells that are found to be normal in shape when a semen analysis is done.

mosaicism   A genetic abnormality in which some cells in the body include a genetic error and other cells have normal genes.

motility   Refers to the movement of the sperm, often measured as the percentage of sperm cells that are moving when a semen analysis is done.

mumps orchitis   An inflammation of the testicle caused by the mumps virus, which can sometimes permanently scar the sperm-producing tissue, causing infertility.

natural cycle IVF   A form of in vitro fertilization in which a woman is given little or no hormone stimulation, and the oocytes that mature in the course of her natural menstrual cycle are harvested transvaginally and fertilized in the laboratory to create embryos for future uterine transfer.

neural tube defect   A problem, such as spina bifida or anencephaly, in which the central nervous system is not developing properly.

nitric oxide   A chemical that acts to transmit messages from one nerve cell to another within the soft tissue of the penis. It is important in the process of erection.

normozoospermic   Having a normal semen analysis.

nucleus   The center of a cell, containing the chromosomes.

oligoasthenoteratozoospermic   Having low sperm concentration and motility, as well as abnormal morphology.

oligozoospermic   Having a low sperm concentration.

oocytes   The eggs produced by a woman's ovary.

open adoption   A model of adoption in which the birth mother and the adoptive parents meet and may have continued contacts over the years with each other and the adopted child.

open biopsy   Taking a sample of tissue in a surgical procedure that involves an incision.

ovarian hyperstimulation syndrome   A medical complication of in vitro fertilization in which the ovaries get so much hormonal stimulation that they swell dangerously and fluid may start filling the pelvic area, affecting respiration.

parent cells   Cells that migrate into the scrotum during fetal development and later produce ripe sperm cells.

parental investment   The amount of energy each parent has to provide in order to ensure that reproduction will occur and that the offspring will survive to adulthood. In humans, females have a higher parental investment than males do.

percutaneous umbilical blood sampling (PUBS)   At weeks 16 to 20 of pregnancy, ultrasound guidance is used to put a needle into the umbilical cord and draw a sample of fetal blood for diagnostic testing.

perivitelline space   An area just inside the zona pellucida of the mature oocyte.

pituitary   A small gland at the base of the brain that produces hormones that control sperm cell production in the testicles.

polymerase chain reaction (PCR)   A laboratory technique used in genetic testing to create many copies of a gene for analysis.

postcoital test   A test in which a couple is asked to have intercourse and then come within a couple of hours to the lab, where the mucus covering the woman's cervix is removed and examined to see whether it contains an adequate number of live sperm cells.

preimplantation genetic diagnosis   Biopsying one or a few cells from an embryo to perform genetic testing and diagnose a problem. It is used to choose normal embryos to transfer in the next stage of in vitro fertilization (IVF).

prolactin   A hormone produced by the pituitary gland that affects milk production in women and also plays a role in sperm production.

prostate   A walnut-sized gland located just under the urinary bladder that produces some of the seminal fluid.

putative father registry   A list of men who think they fathered a child that may be given up for adoption. The putative father can register his interest in the child and be informed of any legal action involving that child.

reactive oxygen species (ROS)   Chemicals that are by-products of oxidation in sperm cells and white blood cells. A high number may signal infection or inflammation.

reproductive fitness   A sociobiological concept that measures biological fitness by the number of one's offspring that survive to reproduce in their own turn.

resuspension   The process in which sperm cells are separated from a larger semen sample and put into a nutrient fluid.

rete testis   Area of the testicle in which sperm cells from the seminiferous tubules collect.

retrograde ejaculation   The condition in which semen takes the path of least resistance when ejaculation begins, spurting backward into the bladder instead of out the tip of the penis.

retroperitoneal lymph node dissection   A surgical procedure done in the course of treating some men who have testicular cancer that can damage nerves involved in controlling ejaculation of semen.

Robertsonian translocation   A condition in which the shorter halves of two different, unpaired chromosomes get lost during cell division, and the longer halves of the two chromosomes fuse together. Since only minor genes are lost, the person with the translocation is healthy. That person's offspring may end up with missing genes or extra ones, however.

semen volume   The amount of seminal fluid in the ejaculate, measured in milliliters (5 ml equals a teaspoon).

seminal plasma   The fluid that makes up semen.

seminal vesicles   Pouchlike glands that sit behind the urinary bladder and produce most of the seminal fluid.

seminiferous tubules   Tiny tubes of tissue in the testicles in which sperm production takes place.

Sertoli cell only syndrome   A finding on testicular biopsy that the sperm-producing tissue of the testis only contains Sertoli cells and no sperm-producing cells.

Sertoli cells   Cells contained in the seminiferous tubules that create a barrier between the bloodstream and the testicle and control the process of sperm production, supplying crucial chemicals that sperm cells need in order to develop.

somatic nerves   The nerves that control sensation and the striated muscles of the body (i.e., the muscles that control movement).

sonogram   An image of part of the body created using sound waves.

sperm concentration   The number of sperm cells found in one milliliter of seminal fluid.

sperm count   The sperm concentration multiplied by the number of milliliters of semen in the sample.

sperm penetration assay (SPA)   A technique in which hamster eggs, with their zona pellucida removed, are put into an incubation dish with specially prepared human sperm cells. The test measures how many eggs are penetrated.

sperm separation   Any of several techniques used to isolate the most motile sperm in the laboratory, for use in assisted reproductive procedures.

spermatids   The next stage in sperm cell development after the spermatocytes divide. Round spermatids have been used to create pregnancies with in vitro fertilization using intracytoplasmic sperm injection.

spermatocytes   A stage in the development of sperm cells in which spermatogonia divide to produce two spermatocytes, each containing only 23 chromosomes.

spermatogonia   A stage in the development of sperm cells in which the stem cell divides to produce two round cells that also each have 46 chromosomes.

spongy body   The lower chamber running down the shaft of the penis, containing the urethra, and expanding to become the glans.

straws   Small, hollow containers used for freezing semen samples.

stricture   A tight band of scar tissue in the urethra that interferes with the free flow of urine and semen.

superovulation   An infertility treatment that combines intrauterine insemination with giving the woman hormones to stimulate her ovaries to produce multiple oocytes.

swim-up   A technique to separate the most motile sperm by having them swim out of the semen into a less dense liquid medium.

sympathetic nerves   Part of the involuntary nervous system, these nerves control the smooth muscle of the prostate and seminal vesicles and the process of emission.

sympathomimetic drugs   Medications that stimulate the sympathetic nerves. These are used to try to provoke normal ejaculation in some men with dry ejaculations.

teratozoospermic   Having abnormally shaped sperm.

testicular sperm extraction (TESE)   A procedure in which sperm cells are isolated by mincing up tissue from a testicular biopsy and using sperm separation techniques.

testosterone   The male sex hormone, produced by the testicles and needed for sperm cell production, puberty, and sexual function.

transurethral resection of the prostate (TURP)   A surgery performed through the urethra, without an incision, to core out an enlarged prostate.

transvaginal ultrasound-guided follicle aspiration   An outpatient procedure that is part of in vitro fertilization and involves using an ultrasound image of the ovaries to guide a needle through the upper vagina into each follicle to aspirate the fluid and oocyte inside.

transvenous embolization   A method in which an interventional radiologist using a fluoroscope X ray can pass a small catheter into a blood vessel, such as a varicocele, and place a coil or balloon in the vessel to block abnormal blood flow. This is an effective way of treating a varicocele.

trimester   Any of the three 13-week periods into which the 39 weeks of a human pregnancy are divided.

triple screen   A blood test of the mother at around week 15 of pregnancy to measure levels of three chemicals: alpha-fetoprotein, unconjugated estriol, and human chorionic gonadotropin. If the test is abnormal, the fetus may have Down syndrome or a neural tube defect.

tunica albuginea   A thick, strong covering of tissue that surrounds the seminiferous tubules within the testicle.

urethra   The tube from the bladder to the opening at the end of the penis that carries urine and semen.

urethritis   An inflammation of the urethra, often from a sexually transmitted disease.

varicocele   A cluster of large, dilated veins that drain blood away from one or both of the testicles, often associated with poor semen quality.

vas deferens   The pair of tubes that transport mature sperm cells from the epididymis to the area where semen is mixed together.

vasoepididymostomy   A microsurgical operation used to connect one end of the vas deferens to a tiny opening created in the epididymis.

vasogram   A special X ray of the sperm pathways, usually done as part of reconstructive surgery.

vasovasostomy   A microsurgical operation used to reconnect the two ends of the vas deferens; for example, to repair a previous vasectomy.

velocity   The speed of sperm movement.

zona-free hamster oocyte penetration assay   See *sperm penetration assay (SPA)*.

zona pellucida   A shell of protein that surrounds the oocyte.

zygote   The fertilized oocyte.

zygote intrafallopian transfer (ZIFT)   An assisted reproductive procedure in which an embryo created in the laboratory is inserted into the fallopian tube rather than through the cervix and into the uterus.

Resources

Infertility Organizations

American Society for Reproductive Medicine (ASRM), 1209 Montgomery Highway, Birmingham, AL 35216-2809; phone: 205-978-5000; fax: 205-978-5005; e-mail: asrm@asrm.com; URL: http://www.asrm.com. ASRM is a society for medical professionals who treat infertility. It offers a variety of support services for patients including informational brochures (For example: *IVF and GIFT: A Guide to Assisted Reproductive Technologies: A Guide for Patients,* 1995), a directory of medical professionals on its web site, updates on infertility news, access to the annual SART reports of assisted reproductive technology (ART) clinic success rates, and a list of state insurance laws relevant to infertility.

American Society of Andrology, URL: http://godot.urol.uic.edu/~androlog/. This organization mainly provides information for professionals involved in studying and treating problems with male reproduction. Their web site includes a very nice reference work, however, *The Handbook of Andrology.* Although this online book, published in 1995, is written for physicians and scientists, you may find it contains some helpful information.

InterNational Council on Infertility Information Dissemination (INCIID), P.O. Box 6836, Arlington, VA 22206; phone: 703-379-9178; fax: 703-379-1593; e-mail: INCIIDinfo@inciid.org.; URL: http://www.inciid.org. This nonprofit organization's mission is to serve as a clearinghouse for information for people with infertility. Their web site is very extensive, with referrals, chat lines on a variety of topics, and links to other sites.

Resolve Inc., 1310 Broadway, Somerville, MA 02144-1779; business phone: 617-623-1156; National Help-Line: 617-623-0744; fax: 617-623-0252; e-mail: resolveinc@aol.com; URL: http://www.resolve.org. Resolve is the national organization supporting couples with infertility. They publish a newsletter and other educational materials. Members can join local support groups or a Member-to-Member network. The Help-Line offers information over the phone. Resolve offers physician referrals and access to the annual SART reports of ART clinic success rates. Resolve advocates for legislation to improve insurance coverage for infertility.

Society for Assisted Reproductive Technology (SART) is an affiliate of the American Society for Reproductive Medicine (see entry above) and can be contacted at the ASRM address and phone number. Each year, SART, in cooperation with the Centers for Disease Control and Prevention (CDC), ASRM, and Resolve (see above), produces a report on ART clinic success rates. The report allows you to search by region or for a specific clinic. You can view the report on line at URL: http://www.cdc.gov/nccdphp/drh/arts/index.htm, call a toll-free number (888-299-1585) for a hard copy of the report, or obtain it through ASRM or Resolve (see above).

Adoption Organizations

Adoptive Families of America, 3333 Highway 100, North Minneapolis, MN 55422; phone: 612-535-4829, 800-372-3300 (toll free); fax: 612-535-7808. URL: http://www.AdoptiveFam.org. A support organization for families considering adoption or who have adopted, Adoptive Families of America offers educational materials and many services.

American Academy of Adoption Attorneys, P.O. Box 33053, Washington, D.C. 20033-0053; phone: 202-832-2222; e-mail: trustees@adoptionattorneys.org; URL: http://www.adoptionattorneys.org. This national association of attorneys in the field of adoption promotes reform in adoption law and gives information on adoption practices.

National Adoption Information Clearinghouse, P.O. Box 1182, Washington, DC 20013-1182; phone: 703-352-3488; 888-251-0075 (toll free); URL: http://www.adoption.com. This group offers information on adoption.

National Council for Adoption, 1930 Seventeenth St. NW, Washington, DC 20009; phone: 202-328-1200. This organization offers information on adoption.

Donor Insemination

Alliance for Donor Insemination Families (Susan Hollander, Ph.D., executive director), 9678 E. Arapahoe Rd., #143, Englewood, CO 80112-3704; phone: 303-220-8400; e-mail: AllianceDI@aol.com. This group offers information and support for DI families.

DI Network, Box 265, Sheffield, S3 7YX, United Kingdom; 101603.2644 @compuserve.com; URL: http://www.issue.co.uk/dinet. This is an international support organization for DI families.

Infertility Insurance

For information on state laws, see American Society for Reproductive Medicine (ASRM) on page 255.

Organon insurance hot line: 800-IVF-PALS (800-483-7257). This hot line provides data on coverage of infertility medications, information on choosing a pharmacy, how to submit claims, and deal with insurance denials. You will need your vital statistics, physician, and insurance plan information to get help from them.

Sperm Banking

American Association of Tissue Banks (AATB), Reproductive Council, 1350 Beverly Rd., Suite 220A, McLean, VA 22101; phone: 707-827-9582; fax: 703-356-2198. The AATB can provide consumer information about sperm bank regulation and a list of sperm banks that have passed their accreditation process. We mention two sperm banks below, not as an endorsement of their quality, but because they offer a large and innovative range of services:

California Cryobank, phone: 800-231-3373; URL: http://www.cryobank.com. This large sperm bank is AATB accredited and has pioneered a range of services, including a donor catalog on their web site.

Xytex Corporation, 1100 Emmett St., Augusta, GA 30904; phone: 706-733-0130; fax: 706-736-9720; e-mail: info@xytex.com; URL: http://www.xytex.com. This network of affiliated sperm banks is not AATB accredited, but it has pioneered giving more detailed information about donors.

Support for Families with Multiple Births

Triplet Connection, P.O. Box 99571, Stockton, CA 95209; phone: 209-474-0885; fax: 209-474-2233; e-mail: tc@tripletconnection.org; URL: http://www.tripletconnection.org. This is a national support organization for families experiencing multiple births (triplets or more). They publish a newsletter, a catalog of products, and more.

Organizations with Directories of Sex Therapists

American Association of Sex Educators, Counselors, and Therapists (AASECT), 435 North Michigan Ave., Suite 1717, Chicago, IL 60611; phone: 312-644-0828.

Society for Sex Therapy and Research (SSTAR); contact SSTAR president Peter Fagan, Ph.D., Sexual Behaviors Consultation Unit, 550 North Broadway, Suite 114, Baltimore, MD 21205; phone: 410-955-6318.

Genetic Testing and Counseling

Alliance of Genetic Support Groups, 35 Wisconsin Circle, Suite 440, Chevy Chase, MD 20815; phone: 800-336-GENE. This alliance provides information on support groups for families with specific genetic problems.

National Society of Genetic Counselors, 233 Canterbury Drive, Wallingford, PA 19086; phone: 610-872-7608. The society can help you find genetic resources in your area.

Books on Infertility

To see a catalogue specializing in books on infertility and adoption, try *Tapestry Books,* P.O. Box 359, Ringoes, NJ 08551; phone: 800-765-2367; fax: 908-788-2999; e-mail: info@tapestrybooks.com; URL: http://webcom.com/tapestry.

Infertility and Cancer
Schover, L. R. 1997. *Sexuality and Infertility after Cancer.* New York: John Wiley & Sons.

Donor Insemination
Vercollone, C. F., Moss, H., and Moss, R. 1997. *Helping the Stork: The Choices and Challenges of Donor Insemination.* New York: Macmillan.

Children's Books
Gordon, E. *Mommy, Did I Grow in Your Tummy?* 1992. Santa Monica, Calif.: E. M. Greenberg Press. (Available from publisher, 1460 Seventh St., Suite 301, Santa Monica, CA 90401.) Reviews ART for young children.

How I Began. 1998. Available from the national office of Resolve (see page 255 for address) or directly from the Fertility Society of Australia, The Royal Women's Hospital, 132 Grattan St., Carlton, Victoria 3053, Australia. Provides information about sperm donation for young children.

Infertility Research Trust. 1991. *My Story.* Sheffield, U.K: J. W. Northend. Available from Kris Probasco, ACSW, 144 Westwoods Drive, Liberty, MO 64068. Story of donor insemination for young children, written in England.

Schaffer, P. 1988. *How Babies and Families Are Made.* Berkeley, Calif.: Tabor Sarah Books. (Available from the publisher, 2419 Jefferson, Berkeley, CA 94703.) Reviews a variety of ways of building families for young children; multiculturally sensitive.

Schnitter, J. 1995. *Let Me Explain: A Story about Donor Insemination.* Indianapolis: Perspectives Press. A great picture book about donor insemination for school-age children.

Male Sexuality
Zilbergeld, B. 1992. *The New Male Sexuality.* New York: Bantam.

Chapter Sources

1. Male Infertility: Bumping into the Iceberg

Statistics on the Prevalence of Infertility

Stephen, E. H. 1996. Projections of impaired fecundity among women in the United States: 1995–2020. *Fertility and Sterility* 66:205–209.

Stephen, E. H., and Chandra, A. 1998. Updated projections of infertility in the United States: 1995–2025. *Fertility and Sterility* 70:30–34.

Decreases over Time in Men's Sperm Counts

Carlsen, E., Gwiercman, A., Keiding, N., and Skakkebaek, N. E. 1992. Evidence for decreasing quality of semen during past 50 years. *British Medical Journal* 305:609–613.

Becker, S., and Berhane, K. 1997. A meta-analysis of 61 sperm count studies revisited. *Fertility and Sterility* 67:1103–1108.

Statistics on the Numbers of Couples Seeking Help for Infertility

Olsen, J., Kuppers-Chinnow, M., and Spinelli, A. 1996. Seeking medical help for subfecundity: A study based upon surveys in five European countries. *Fertility and Sterility* 66:95–100.

Wilcox, L. S., and Mosher, W. D. 1993. Use of infertility services in the United States. *Obstetrics and Gynecology* 82:122–127.

Effectiveness of ICSI

Sherins, R. J., Thorsell, L. P., Dorfmann A., et al. 1995. Intracytoplasmic sperm injection facilitates fertilization even in the most severe forms of male infertility: Pregnancy outcome correlates with maternal age and number of eggs available. *Fertility and Sterility* 64:369–375.

Tournaye, H., Liu, J., Nagy, Z., et al. 1995. Intracytoplasmic sperm injection (ICSI): The Brussels experience. *Reproductive Fertility and Development* 7:269–279.

2. Getting Started with a Male Infertility Workup

Statistics on Specialists in the American Society for Reproductive Medicine
ASRM Web Site. 1998. http://www.asrm.com. Accessed August 31.

Missing a General Health Problem Related to Male Infertility
Jarow, J. P. 1994. Life-threatening conditions associated with male infertility. *Urologic Clinics of North America* 21:409–415.

3. They Want Me to Go into a Little Room and Do *What?*

Semen Quality Deteriorates if No Ejaculation
Pellestor, F., Girardet, A., and Andreo, B. 1994. Effect of long abstinence periods on human sperm quality. *International Journal of Fertility and Menopausal Studies* 39:278–282.

Better Semen Samples with an Erotic Video
Van Roijen, J. H., Slob, A. K., Gianotten, W. L., Dohle, G. R., van der Zon, A. T., Vreeburg, J. T., and Weber, R. F. 1996. Sexual arousal and the quality of semen produced by masturbation. *Human Reproduction* 11:147–151.

Jewish Views on Masturbation to Collect Semen
Schenker, J. G. 1996. Infertility evaluation and treatment according to Jewish law. *European Association of Gynaecologists and Obstetricians Newsletter* 2(2):1–13.

Islamic Views on Masturbation to Collect Semen
Serour, G. I. 1996. Bioethics in infertility management in the Muslim World. *European Association of Gynaecologists and Obstetricians Newsletter* 2(2):1–7.

Roman Catholic Views on Masturbation to Collect Semen
Sparks, R. C. 1997. Helping childless couples conceive. St. Anthony's Messenger Online, http://www.americancatholic.org/messenger/0497/feature1.html. Accessed December 3.

Protestant Views on Masturbation to Collect Semen
Dunstan, G. R. 1996. Christian moral reasoning. *European Association of Gynaecologists and Obstetricians Newsletter* 2(2):1–5.

Semen Quality from Intercourse versus Masturbation
Sofikitis, N. V., and Miyagawa, I. 1993. Endocrinological, biophysical, and biochemical parameters of semen collected via masturbation versus sexual intercourse. *Journal of Andrology* 14:366–373.

4. Your Baby-Making Machinery: An Owner's Manual

General Information on Sperm Development and Anatomy
Lipshultz, L. I., and Howards, S. S. eds. 1997. *Infertility in the Male* (3rd ed.). St. Louis: Mosby–Year Book.

Numbers of Sperm That Reach Their Goal
Settlage, D. S., Motoshima, M., and Tredway, D. R. 1973. Sperm transport from the external cervical os to the fallopian tubes in women: A time and quantitation study. *Fertility and Sterility* 24:655–661.

A More Recent Study of Sperm Numbers
Williams, M., Hill, C.J., Scudamore, I., Dunphy, B., Cooke, I. D., and Barratt, C. L. 1993. Sperm numbers and distribution within the human fallopian tube around ovulation. *Human Reproduction* 8:2019–2026.

Sonograms of Sperm Transport through the Uterus
Kunz, G., Beil, D., Deininger, H., Wildt, L., and Leyendecker, G. 1996. The dynamics of rapid sperm transport through the female genital tract: Evidence from vaginal sonography of uterine peristalsis and hysterosalpingoscintigraphy. *Human Reproduction* 11:627–632.

Sperm Competition
Baker, R. R., and Bellis, M. A. 1995. *Human Sperm Competition: Copulation, Masturbation and Infidelity.* London: Chapman & Hall.

Baker, R. R. 1996. *Sperm Wars: The Science of Sex.* New York: Basic Books.

Pregnancy Rates in Fertile Couples
Zinaman, M. J., Clegg, E. D., Brown, C. C., O'Connor, J., and Selevan, S. G. 1996. Estimates of human fertility and pregnancy loss. *Fertility and Sterility* 65:503–509.

Pregnancy Rates in Untreated Infertile Couples
Collins, J. A., Burrows, E. A., and Willan, A. R. 1995. The prognosis for live birth among untreated infertile couples. *Fertility and Sterility* 64:22–28.

5. The Semen Analysis and Other Diagnostic Tests for Male Infertility

The Semen Analysis
Overstreet, J. W., and Brazil, C. 1997. Semen analysis. In *Infertility in the Male* (3rd ed.), edited by L. I. Lipshultz and S. S. Howards. St. Louis: Mosby–Year Book, 487–490.

Specialized Tests of Sperm Function
Tripp, B. M., Gagnon, C. 1997. Advanced sperm fertility tests. In *Infertility in the Male* (3rd ed.), edited by L. I. Lipshultz and S. S. Howards. St. Louis: Mosby–Year Book, 194–209.

Specialized Physical Examinations
Coburn, M., Kim, E. D., and Wheeler, T. M. 1997. Testicular biopsy in male infertility evaluation. In *Infertility in the Male* (3rd ed.), edited by L. I. Lipshultz and S. S. Howards. St. Louis: Mosby–Year Book, 219–248.

6. Starting the Production Line: Sex and Fertility

Sexual Desire
Segraves, R. T. Hormones and libido. In *Sexual Desire Disorders,* edited by S. R. Leiblum and R. C. Rosen. New York: Guilford Press, 271–312.

Mechanics of Erection
Andersson, K. E., and Stief, C. G. 1997. Neurotransmission and the contraction and relaxation of penile erectile tissues. *World Journal of Urology* 15:14–20.

Christ, C. J. 1997. The "syncytial tissue triad": A model for understanding how gap junctions participate in the local control of penile erection. *World Journal of Urology* 15:36–44.

Aging and Erections
Feldman, H. A., Goldstein, I., Hatzichristou, G., Krane, R. J., and McKinlay, J. B. 1994. Impotence and its medical and psychosocial correlates: Results of the Massachusetts Male Aging Study. *Journal of Urology* 151:54–61.

Lubricants and Sperm Cell Damage
Kutteh, W. H., Chao, C. H., Ritter, J. O., and Byrd, W. 1996. Vaginal lubricants for the infertile couple: Effect on sperm activity. *International Journal of Fertility and Menopausal Studies* 41:400–404.

Timing of Intercourse in Relation to Ovulation
Ferreira-Poblete, A. 1997. The probability of conception on different days of the cycle with respect to ovulation: An overview. *Advances in Contraception* 13:83–95.

Wilcox, A. J., Weinberg, C. R., and Baird, D. D. 1995. Timing of sexual intercourse in relation to ovulation: Effects on the probability of conception, survival of the pregnancy, and sex of the baby. *New England Journal of Medicine* 333:1517–1521.

Agarwal, S. K., and Haney, A. F. 1994. Does recommending timed intercourse really help the infertile couple? *Obstetrics and Gynecology* 84:307–310.

Study from Israel on Timing of Intercourse
Tur-Kaspa, I., Maor, Y., Levran, D., Yonish, M., Mashiach, S., and Dor, J. 1994. How often should infertile men have intercourse to achieve conception? *Fertility and Sterility* 62:370–375.

Study of Live Births in Untreated Infertile Couples
Collins, J. A., Burrows, E. A., and Willan, A. R. 1995. The prognosis for live birth among untreated infertile couples. *Fertility and Sterility* 64:22–28.

Sperm Counts and Motility, and Time to Pregnancy
Ayala, C., Steinberger, E., and Smith, D. P. 1996. The influence of semen analysis parameters on the fertility potential of infertile couples. *Journal of Andrology* 17:718–725.

7. Holes in Our Genes: Inherited Causes of Infertility

General References on Genetics and Male Infertility
Jaffe, T., and Oates, R. D. 1997. Genetic aspects of infertility. In *Infertility in the Male* (3rd ed.), edited by L. I. Lipshultz and S. S. Howards. St. Louis: Mosby–Year Book, 280–304.

Johnson, M. D. 1998. Genetic risks of intracytoplasmic sperm injection in the treatment of male infertility: Recommendations for genetic counseling and screening. *Fertility and Sterility* 70:397–411.

Rapid Changes on the Y Chromosome
Radelsky, P. 1997. Y? *Discover* (November): 89–91, 93.

Klinefelter Syndrome and XYY Syndrome
Jorde, L. B., Carey, J. C., and White, R. L. 1995. *Medical Genetics.* St. Louis: Mosby–Year Book, 114–115.

Tournaye, H., Staessen, C., Liebaers, I., et al. 1996. Testicular sperm recovery in nine 47,XXY Klinefelter patients. *Human Reproduction* 11:1644–1649.

Johnson, M. D. 1998. Genetic risks of intracytoplasmic sperm injection in the treatment of male infertility: Recommendations for genetic counseling and screening. *Fertility and Sterility* 70:397–411.

Microdeletions of the Y Chromosome
Pryor, J. L., Kent-First, M., Muallem, A., Van Bergen, A. H., Nolten, W. E., Meisner, L., and Roberts, K. P. 1997. Microdeletions in the Y chromosome of infertile men. *New England Journal of Medicine* 336:534–539.

Reijo, R., Alagappan, R. K., Patrizio, P., and Page, D. C. 1996. Severe oligozoospermia resulting from deletions of azoospermia factor gene on Y chromosome. *Lancet* 347(9011):1290–1293.

Kent-First, M. G., Kol, S., Muallem, A., Ofir, R., Manor, D., Blazer, S., First, N., and Itskovitz-Eldor, J. 1996. The incidence and possible relevance of Y-linked microdeletions in babies born after intracytoplasmic sperm injection and their infertile fathers. *Molecular Human Reproduction* 2:943–950.

Cooke, H. J., Hargreave, T., and Elliot, D. J. 1998. Understanding the genes involved in spermatogenesis: A progress report. *Fertility and Sterility* 69:989–995.

Translocations

Jorde, L. B., Carey, J.C., White, R. L. 1995. *Medical Genetics.* St. Louis: Mosby–Year Book, 117–120.

Wilkins-Haug, L. E., Rein, M. S., and Hornstein, M. D. 1997. Oligospermic men: The role of karyotype analysis prior to intracytoplasmic sperm injection. *Fertility and Sterility* 67:612–614.

Van Assche, E., Bonduelle, M., Tournaye, H., Joris, H., Verheyen, G., Devroey, P., Van Steirteghem, A., and Liebaers, I. 1996. Cytogenetics of infertile men. *Human Reproduction* 11:1–24.

Testart, J., Gautier, E., Brami, C., Rolet, F., Sedbon, E., and Thebault, A. 1996. Intra-cytoplasmic sperm injection in infertile patients with structural chromosome abnormalities. *Human Reproduction* 11:2609–2612.

CBAVD and Mutations of the CFTR Gene

Chillon, M., Casals, T., Mercier, B., Bassas, L., Lissens, W., Silber, S., Romey, M., Ruiz-Romero, J., Verlingue, C., Claustres, M., Nunes, V., Ferec, C., and Estivill, X. 1995. Mutations in the cystic fibrosis gene in patients with congenital absence in the vas deferens. *New England Journal of Medicine* 332:1475–1480.

Lissens, W., Mercier, B., Tournaye, H., Bonduelle, M., Ferec, C., Seneca, S., Devroey, P., Silber, S., Van Steirteghem, A., and Liebaers, I. 1996. Cystic fibrosis and infertility caused by congenital bilateral absence of the vas deferens and related clinical entities. *Human Reproduction* 11 (Suppl.):55–78.

CF Mutations in Men with Abnormal Semen Quality

Van der Ven, K., Messer, L., van der Ven, H., Jeyendran, R. S., and Ober, C. 1996. Cystic fibrosis mutation screening in healthy men with reduced sperm quality. *Human Reproduction* 11:513–517.

Tuerlings, J. H. A. M., Mol, B., Kremer, J. A. M., et al. 1998. Mutation frequency of cystic fibrosis transmembrane regulator is not increased in oligozoospermic male candidates for intracytoplasmic sperm injection. *Fertility and Sterility* 69:899–903.

Immotile Cilia Syndrome

McConnell, J. D. 1997. Abnormalities in sperm motility: Techniques of evaluation and treatment. In *Infertility in the Male* (3rd ed.), edited by L. I. Lipshultz and S. S. Howards. St. Louis: Mosby–Year Book, 249–267.

Abnormal Karyotypes and Microdeletions in Men Having IVF with ICSI

Testart, J., Gautier, E., Brami, C., Rolet, F., Sedbon, E., and Thebault, A. 1996. Intracytoplasmic sperm injection in infertile patients with structural chromosome abnormalities. *Human Reproduction* 11:2609–2612.

Kent-First, M. G., Kol, S., Muallem, A., Ofir, R., Manor, D., Blazer, S., First, N., and Itskovitz-Eldor, J. 1996. The incidence and possible relevance of Y-linked microdeletions in babies born after intracytoplasmic sperm injection and their infertile fathers. *Molecular Human Reproduction* 2:943–950.

Meschede, D., Lemcke, B., Exeler, J. R., et al. 1998. Chromosome abnormalities in 447 couples undergoing intracytoplasmic sperm injection—prevalence, types, sex distribution and reproductive relevance. *Human Reproduction* 13:576–582.

Abnormal Chromosomes in Sperm Cells of Men with Normal Karyotypes

Martin, R. H. 1996. The risk of chromosomal abnormalities following ICSI. *Human Reproduction* 11:924–925.

Genetic Abnormalities in IVF Embryos

Munne, S., Marquez, C., Reing, A., Garrisi, J., and Alikani, M. 1998. Chromosome abnormalities in embryos obtained after conventional in vitro fertilization and intracytoplasmic sperm injection. *Fertility and Sterility* 69:904–908.

Interviews with IVF Couples about Prenatal Diagnosis

Schover, L. R., Thomas, A. J., Falcone, T., Attaran, M., and Goldberg, J. 1998. Attitudes about genetic risk of couples undergoing in vitro fertilization. *Human Reproduction* 13:862–866.

Health of Children Born from IVF-ICSI

Tournaye, H., Liu, J., Nagy, Z., et al. 1995. Intracytoplasmic sperm injection (ICSI): The Brussels experience. *Reproduction, Fertility and Development* 7:269–278.

Aytoz, A., Camus, M., Tournaye, H., et al. 1998. Outcome of pregnancies after intracytoplasmic sperm injection and the effect of sperm origin and quality on this outcome. *Fertility and Sterility* 70:500–505.

Bowen, J. R., Gibson, F. L., Leslie, G. I., and Saunders, D. M. 1998. Medical and developmental outcome at one year for children conceived by intracytoplasmic sperm injection. *Lancet* 351:1529–1534.

Bonduelle, M., Joris, H., Hofman, K., Liebaers, I., and Van Steirteghem, A. 1998. Mental development of 201 ICSI children at 2 years of age. *Lancet* 351:1553.

8. Developmental Problems That Cause Infertilty

Undescended Testicles

Coughlin, M. T., O'Leary, L. A., Songer, N. J., Bellinger, M. F., LaPorte, R. E., and Lee, P. A. 1997. Time to conception after orchidopexy: Evidence for subfertility? *Fertility and Sterility* 67:742–746.

Mandat, K. M., Wieczorkiewicz, B., Gubala-Kacala, M., Sypniewski, J., and Bujok, G. 1994. Semen analysis of patients who had orchidopexy in childhood. *European Journal of Pediatric Surgery* 4:94–97.

Lee, P. A., O'Leary, L. A., Songer, N. J., Bellinger, M. F., and LaPorte, R. E. 1995. Paternity after cryptorchidism: Lack of correlation with age at orchidopexy. *British Journal of Urology* 75:704–707.

Lee, P. A., O'Leary, L. A., Songer, N. J., Coughlin, M. T., Bellinger, M. F., and LaPorte, R. E. 1996. Paternity after unilateral cryptorchidism: A controlled study. *Pediatrics* 98:676–679.

Theory about Environmental Pollutants and Cryptorchidism, Hypospadias, and Testicular Cancer

Petersen, P. M., Gwiercman, A., Skakkebaek, N. E., et al. 1998. Gonadal function in men with testicular cancer. *Seminars in Oncology* 25:224–233.

9. Germs and Germ Cells: Infections and Infertilty

Using Microsurgery to Repair Obstruction after Mumps Orchitis

Sabanegh, E., Jr., and Thomas, A. J., Jr. 1995. Effectiveness of crossover transseptal vasoepididymostomy in treating complex obstructive azoospermia. *Fertility and Sterility* 63:392–395.

Rates of Mumps in United States

Van Loon, F. P., Holmes, S. J., Srotkin, B. L., et al. 1995. Mumps surveillance—United States, 1988-1993. *MMWR CDC Surveillance Summaries* 44:1–14.

Fathering a Child for an HIV-Positive Man

Dussaix, E., Guetard, D., Dauguet, C., et al. 1993. Spermatozoa as potential carriers of HIV. *Research in Virology* 144:487–495.

Marina, S., Marina, F., Alcolea, R., et al. 1998. Human immunodeficiency virus type 1—Serodiscordant couples can bear healthy children after undergoing intrauterine insemination. *Fertility and Sterility* 70:35–39.

STDs, Sperm Counts, and Male Infertility

Ness, R. B., Markovic, N., Carlson, C. L., and Coughlin, M. T. 1997. Do men become infertile after having sexually transmitted urethritis? An epidemiologic examination. *Fertility and Sterility* 68:205–213.

Chlamydia and Female Infertility

Eggert-Kruse, W., Buhlinger-Gopfarth, N., Rohr, G., et al. 1996. Antibodies to chlamydia trachomatis in semen and relationship with parameters of male fertility. *Human Reproduction* 11:1408–1417.

Study of 1,710 Men Tested for White Cells

Yanushpolsky, E. H., Politch, J. A., Hill, J. A., and Anderson, D. J. 1996. Is leukocytospermia clinically relevant? *Fertility and Sterility* 66:822–825.

Antibiotic Treatment Study for White Cells

Yanushpolsky, E. H., Politch, J. A., Hill, J. A., and Anderson, D. J. 1995. Antibiotic therapy and leukocytospermia: A prospective, randomized, controlled study. *Fertility and Sterility* 63:142–147.

Antibiotic Studies with More Positive Results

Erel, C. T., Senturk, L. M., Demir, F., Irez, T., and Ertungealp, E. 1997. Antibiotic therapy in men with leukocytospermia. *International Journal of Fertility and Women's Medicine* 42:206–210.

Yamamoto, M., Hibi, H., Katsuno, S., and Miyake, K. 1995. Antibiotic and ejaculation treatments improve resolution rate of leukocytospermia in infertile men with prostatitis. *Nagoya Journal of Medical Science* 58:41–45.

ROS and Male Infertility

Sharma, R. K., and Agarwal, A. 1996. Role of reactive oxygen species in male infertility. *Urology* 48:835–350.

Vitamins to Reduce ROS

Ford, W. C. L., and Whittington, K. 1998. Antioxidant treatment for male subfertility: A promise that remains unfulfilled. *Human Reproduction* 13:1416–1418.

Tarin, J. J., Brines, J., and Cano, A. 1998. Is antioxidant therapy a promising strategy to improve human reproduction? *Human Reproduction* 13:1415–1416.

Reasons for Formation of Antisperm Antibodies

Gubin, D. A., Dmochowski, R., and Kutteh, W. H. 1998. Multivariant analysis of men from infertile couples with and without antisperm antibodies. *American Journal of Reproductive Immunology* 39:157–160.

Pregnancy Rates with IVF versus IVF-ICSI with Antisperm Antibodies

Lahteenmaki, A., Reima, I., and Hovatta, O. 1995. Treatment of severe male immunological infertility by intracytoplasmic sperm injection. *Human Reproduction* 10:2824–2828.

Mercan, R., Oehninger, S., Muasher, S. J., Toner, J. P., and Mayer, J., Jr., and Lanzendorf, S. E. 1998. Impact of fertilization history and semen parameters on ICSI outcome. *Journal of Assisted Reproduction and Genetics* 15:39–45.

Culligan, P. J., Crane, M. M., Boone, W. R., et al. 1998. Validity and cost-effectiveness of antisperm antibody testing before in vitro fertilization. *Fertility and Sterility* 69:894–898.

10. The Boulder on the Path: Obstructive Infertility

Success of Vasectomy Reversals

Belker, A. M., Thomas, A. J., Jr., Fuchs, E. F., Konnak, J. W., and Sharlip, I. D. 1991. Results of 1,469 microsurgical vasectomy reversals by the Vasovasostomy Study Group. *Journal of Urology* 145:505–511.

11. Is It My Hormones?

Hormones and Male Infertility
Zokol, R. Z., and Swerdloff, R. S. 1997. Endocrine evaluation. In *Infertility in the Male* (3rd ed.), edited by L. I. Lipshultz and S. S. Howards. St. Louis: Mosby–Year Book, 210–218.

Abnormal Sperm Cell Production
Coburn, M., Kim, E. D., and Wheeler, T. M. 1997. Testicular biopsy in male infertility evaluation. In *Infertility in the Male* (3rd ed.), edited by L. I. Lipshultz and S. S. Howards. St. Louis: Mosby–Year Book, 219–248.

12. Varicoceles: How Important Are They?

Varicoceles
Mellinger, B. C. 1995. Varicocelectomy. *Techniques in Urology* 1:188–196.

Thomas, A. J., Jr., and Geisinger, M. A. 1990. Current management of varicoceles. *Urologic Clinics of North America* 17:893–907.

Dewire, D. M., Thomas, A. J., Jr., Falk, R., Geisinger, M. A., and Lammert, G. K. 1994. Clinical outcome and cost comparison of percutaneous embolization and surgical ligation of varicocele. *Journal of Andrology* 15 (Suppl.): 38S–42S.

World Health Organization Study of Varicoceles
World Health Organization. 1992. The influence of varicocele on parameters of fertility in a large group of men presenting to infertility clinics. *Fertility and Sterility* 57:1289–1293.

Study by Israeli Group on Fixing Varicoceles
Madgar, I., Weissenberg, R., Lunenfeld, B., Karasik, A., and Goldwasser, B. 1995. Controlled trial of high spermatic vein ligation for varicocele in infertile men. *Fertility and Sterility* 63:120–124.

Benefits of Embolization of Varicoceles
Dewire, D. M., Thomas, A. J., Jr., Falk, R. M., Geisinger, M. A., and Lammert, G. K. 1994. Clinical outcome and cost comparison of percutaneous embolization and surgical ligation of varicocele. *Journal of Andrology* 15 (Suppl.): 38S–42S.

13. The Dry Ejaculation: Not a Sexual Technique

Retrograde Ejaculation
Okada, H., Fujioka, H., Tatsumi, N., et al. 1998. Treatment of patients with retrograde ejaculation in the era of modern assisted reproduction technology. *Journal of Urology* 159:848–850.

Vibration Stimulation

Ohl, N. A., Sonksen, J., Menge, A. C., McCabe, M., and Keller, L. M. 1997. Electro-ejaculation versus vibratory stimulation in spinal cord injured men: Sperm quality and patient preference. *Journal of Urology* 157:2147–2149.

Electroejaculation

Chung, P. H., Yeko, T. R., Mayer, J. C., Sanford, E. J., and Maroulis, G. B. 1995. Assisted fertility using electroejaculation in men with spinal cord injury: A review of literature. *Fertility and Sterility* 64:1–9.

14. Adding Insult to Injury: Infertility after Cancer Treatment

General Reference for Infertility after Cancer

Schover, L. R. 1997. *Sexuality and Infertility after Cancer.* New York: John Wiley & Sons.

Fertility after Chemotherapy with Cis-platinum

Pont, J., and Albrecht, W. 1997. Fertility after chemotherapy for testicular germ cell cancer. *Fertility and Sterility* 68:1–5.

Fertility after Bone Marrow Transplantation

Chatterjee, R., and Goldstone, A. H. 1996. Gonadal damage and effects on fertility in adult patients with haematological malignancy undergoing stem cell trans-plantation. *Bone Marrow Transplantation* 17:5–11.

Cleveland Clinic Study on Banking Sperm before Cancer

Agarwal, A., Sidhu, R. K., Shekarriz, M., and Thomas, A. J. 1995. Optimum absti-nence time for cryopreservation of semen in cancer patients. *Journal of Urol-ogy* 154:86–88.

Sperm Banking for Teenagers

Kliesch, S., Behre, H. M., Jurgens, H., and Nieschlag, E. 1996. Cryopreservation of semen from adolescent patients with malignancies. *Medical and Pediatric Oncology* 26:20–27.

Schover, L. R., Agarwal, A., and Thomas, A. T. 1998. Cryopreservation of gametes in young patients with cancer. *Journal of Pediatric Hematology/Oncology* 5:426–428.

Cost of Sperm Banking

Meistrich, M. L., Vassilopoulou-Sellin, R., and Lipshultz, L. I. 1997. Gonadal dys-function. In *Cancer: Principles and Practice of Oncology* (5th ed.), edited by V. T. Devita, S. Hellman, and S. A. Rosenberg. Philadelphia: Lippincott-Raven, 2758–2773.

15. Does Lifestyle Contribute to Male Infertility?

Exercise and Testosterone Production
Mantzoros, C. S., and Georgiadis, E. I. 1995. Body mass and physical activity are important predictors of serum androgen concentrations in young healthy men. *Epidemiology* 6:432–435.

No Advantage of Boxer Shorts
Tiemessen, C. H. J., Evers, J. L., and Bots, R. S. G. M. 1995. Tight fitting underwear and sperm quality. *Lancet* 347:1844–1845.

The Testicular Hypothermia Device
Zorgniotti, A., Cohen, M., and Sealfon, A. 1986. Chronic scrotal hypothermia: Results in 90 infertile couples. *Journal of Urology* 135:944–948.

Saunas and Fertility
Lähdetie, J. 1995. Occupation- and exposure-related studies on human sperm. *Journal of Occupational and Environmental Medicine* 37:922–930.

Smoking and Fertility
Vine, M. F. 1996. Smoking and male reproduction: A review. *International Journal of Andrology* 19:323–337.

Hughes, E. G., and Brennan, B. G. 1996. Does cigarette smoking impair natural or assisted fecundity? *Fertility and Sterility* 66:679–689.

Close, C. E., Roberts, P. L., and Berger, R. E. 1990. Cigarettes, alcohol and marijuana are related to pyospermia in infertile men. *Journal of Urology* 144:900–903.

Alcohol and Fertility
Olsen, J., Bolumar, F., Boldsen, J., and Bisanti, L. 1997. Does moderate alcohol intake reduce fecundability? A European multicenter study on infertility and subfecundity. *Alcoholism, Clinical and Experimental Research* 21:206–212.

Goverde, H. J., Dekker, H. S., Janssen, H. J., et al. 1995. Semen quality and frequency of smoking and alcohol consumption—An explorative study. *International Journal of Fertility and Menopausal Studies* 40:135–138.

Caffeine and Fertility
Bolumar, F., Olsen, J., Rebagliato, M., and Bisanti, L. 1997. Caffeine intake and delayed conception: A European multicenter study on infertility and subfecundity. *American Journal of Epidemiology* 145:324–334.

Parazzini, F., Marchini, M., Tozzi, L., Messopane, R., and Fedele, L. 1993. Risk factors for unexplained dyspermia in infertile men: A case-control study. *Archives of Andrology* 31:105–113.

Recreational Drugs and Male Infertility
Close, C. E., Roberts, P. L., and Berger, R. E. 1990. Cigarettes, alcohol and marijuana are related to pyospermia in infertile men. *Journal of Urology* 144:900–903.

Li, H., George, V. K., Bianco, F. J., Jr., Lawrence, W. D., and Dhabuwala, C. B. 1997. Histopathological changes in the testes of prepubertal male rats after chronic administration of cocaine. *Journal of Environmental Pathology, Toxicology and Oncology* 16:67–71.

Psychological Stress and Male Infertility

Schenker, J. G., Meirow, D., and Schenker, E. 1992. Stress and human reproduction. *European Journal of Obstetrics, Gynecology, and Reproductive Biology* 45:1–8.

Fenster, L., Katz, D. F., Wyrobek, A. J., et al. 1997. Effects of psychological stress on human semen quality. *Journal of Andrology* 18:194–202.

Drudy, L., Harrison, R., Verso, J., et al. 1994. Does patient semen quality alter during an in vitro fertilization (IVF) program in a manner that is clinically significant when specific counseling is in operation? *Journal of Assisted Reproduction and Genetics* 11:185–188.

Ragni, G., Carramo, A. 1992. Negative effect of stress of in vitro fertilization program on quality of semen. *Acta Europaea Fertilitatis* 23:21–23.

Occupational Factors and Male Fertility

U.S. Department of Health and Human Services. *Reproductive Hazards in the Workplace: Bibliography.*

Lähdetie, J. 1995. Occupation- and exposure-related studies on human sperm. *Journal of Occupational and Environmental Medicine* 37:922–930.

De Cock, J., Westveer, K., Heederik, D., te Velde, D., and van Kooij, R. 1994. Time to pregnancy and occupational exposure to pesticides in fruit growers in the Netherlands. *Occupational and Environmental Medicine* 51: 693–699.

Lin, S., Hwang, S. A., Marshall, E. G., Stone, R., and Chen, J. 1996. Fertility rates among lead workers and professional bus drivers: A comparative study. *Annals of Epidemiology* 6:201–218.

Figa-Talamanca, I., Cini, C., Varricchio, G. C., et al. 1996. Effects of prolonged auto vehicle driving on male reproduction function: A study among taxi drivers. *American Journal of Industrial Medicine* 30:750–758.

Decline in Sperm Counts

Becker, S., and Berhane, K. 1997. A meta-analysis of 61 sperm count studies revisited. *Fertility and Sterility* 67:1103–1108.

Younglai, E. V., Collins, J. A., and Foster, W. G. 1998. Canadian semen quality: An analysis of sperm density among eleven academic fertility centers. *Fertility and Sterility* 70:76–80.

Vierula, M., Niemi, M., Keiski, A., et al. 1996. High and unchanged sperm counts of Finnish men. *International Journal of Andrology* 19:11–17.

Joffe, M. 1996. Decreased fertility in Britain compared with Finland. *Lancet* 347(9014):1519–1522.

Daston, G. P., Gooch, J. W., Breslin, W. J., et al. 1997. Environmental estrogens and reproductive health: A discussion of the human and environmental data. *Reproductive Toxicology* 11:465–481.

Adlercreutz, H., and Mazur, W. 1997. Phyto-oestrogens and Western diseases. *Annals of Medicine* 29:95–120.

16. Using Assisted Reproductive Technology to Treat Male Infertility

Success of IUI

Gilbaugh, J. H., III. 1997. Intrauterine insemination. In *Infertility in the Male* (3rd ed.), edited by L. I. Lipshultz and S. S. Howards. St. Louis: Mosby–Year Book, 439–449.

Success Rates with ICSI

SART report for 1995, http://www.cdc.gove/nccdphp/drh/arts/fig13.htm, accessed July 24, 1998.

Religious Attitudes to ART

Sparks, R. C. 1997. Helping childless couples conceive. St. Anthony's Messenger Online. http://www.americancatholic.org/messenger/0497/feature1.html, accessed December 3.

Dunstan, G. R. 1996. Christian moral reasoning. *European Association of Gynaecologists and Obstetricians Newsletter* 2(2):1–5.

Schenker, J. G. 1996. Infertility evaluation and treatment according to Jewish law. *European Association of Gynaecologists and Obstetricians Newsletter* 2(2):1–13.

Schwartz, A. 1994. A rabbinic response to infertility. In *Be Fruitful and Multiply: Fertility Therapy and the Jewish Tradition*, edited by R. V. Graz. Jerusalem: Genesis Jerusalem Press.

Serour, G. I. 1996. Bioethics in infertility management in the Muslim World. *European Association of Gynaecologists and Obstetricians Newsletter* 2(2):1–7.

Depression and Failure to Get Pregnant

Domar, A. D., Zuttermeister, O. C., Seibel, M., and Benson, H. 1992. Psychological improvement in infertile women after behavioral treatment: A replication. *Fertility and Sterility* 58:144–147.

Schenker, J. G., Meirow, D., and Schenker, E. 1992. Stress and human reproduction. *European Journal of Obstetrics and Gynecology and Reproductive Biology* 45:1–8.

Overall Levels of Distress in Couples with Infertility

Greil, A. L. 1997. Infertility and psychological distress: A critical review. *Social Science and Medicine* 45:1679–1704.

Careful Study of Mood and Success of IVF

Boivin, J., and Takefman, J. E. 1995. Stress level across stages of in vitro fertilization in subsequently pregnant and nonpregnant women. *Fertility and Sterility* 64:801–810.

Pregnancy as a Result of Rape

Holmes, M. M., Resnick, H. S., Kilpatrick, D. G., and Best, C. L. 1996. Rape-related pregnancy: Estimates and descriptive characteristics from a national sample of women. *American Journal of Obstetrics and Gynecology* 175:320–324.

Evidence That Stress May Contribute to Early Miscarriage

Neugebauer, R., Kline, J., Stein, Z., Shrout, P., Warburton, D., and Susser, M. 1996. Association of stressful life events with chromosomally normal spontaneous abortions. *American Journal of Epidemiology* 143:588–596.

O'Hare, T., and Creed, F. 1995. Life events and miscarriage: *British Journal of Psychiatry* 167:799–805.

Stress May Contribute to Poor Health During Pregnancy

Rostad, B., Schei, B., and Jacobsen, G. 1995. Health consequences of severe life events for pregnancy. *Scandinavian Journal of Primary Health Care* 13:99–104.

Stress During IVF Is Not Striking

Boivin, J., Takefman, J. E. 1996. Impact of the in-vitro fertilization process on emotional, physical and relational variables. *Human Reproduction* 11:903–907.

Boivin, J. 1997. Is there too much emphasis on psychosocial counseling for infertile patients? *Journal of Assisted Reproduction and Genetics* 14:184–186.

Excess Optimism about Pregnancy Rates

Leiblum, S. R., Kemmann, E., and Lane, M. K. 1987. The psychological concomitants of in vitro fertilization. *Journal of Psychosomatic Obstetrics and Gynaecology* 6:165–178.

Hearn, M. T., Yuzpe, A. A., Brown, S. E., and Casper, R. F. 1987. Psychological characteristics of in vitro fertilization participants. *American Journal of Obstetrics and Gynecology,* 156:269–274.

Emotional Reaction to Failed IVF

Baram, D., Tourtelot, E., Muechler, E., and Huang, K. 1988. Psychosocial adjustment following unsuccessful in vitro fertilization. *Journal of Psychosomatic Obstetrics and Gynaecology* 9:181–190.

Litt, M. D., Tennen, H., Affleck, G., Klock, S. 1992. Coping and cognitive factors in adaptation to in vitro fertilization failure. *Journal of Behavioral Medicine* 15:171–186.

Newton, C. R., Hearn, M. T., and Yuzpe, A. A. 1990. Psychological assessment and follow-up after in vitro fertilization: Assessing the impact of failure. *Fertility and Sterility* 54:879–886.

Multiple Births and ART

Wilcox, L. S., Kiely, J. L., Melvin, C. L., and Martin, M. C. 1996. Assisted reproductive technologies: Estimates of their contribution to multiple births and newborn hospital days in the United States. *Fertility and Sterility* 65:361–366.

Doyle, P. 1996. The outcome of multiple pregnancy. *Human Reproduction* 11(Suppl. 4):110–117.

ART Couples' Attitudes to Multiple Births

Gleicher, N., Campbell, D. P., Chan, C. L., et al. 1995. The desire for multiple births in couples with infertility problems contradicts present practice patterns. *Human Reproduction* 10:1079–1084.

Goldfarb, J., Kinzer, D. J., Boyle, M., and Kurit, D. 1996. Attitudes of in vitro fertilization and intrauterine insemination couples toward multiple gestation pregnancy and multifetal pregnancy reduction. *Fertility and Sterility* 65:815–820.

Fetal Reduction Improves the Outcome of Triplet Pregnancies

Smith-Levitin, M., Kowalik, A., Birnholz, J., et al. 1996. Selective reduction of multifetal pregnancies to twins improves outcome over nonreduced triplet gestations. *American Journal of Obstetrics and Gynecology* 175:878–892.

Souter, I., and Goodwin, T. M. 1998. Decision making in multifetal pregnancy reduction for triplets. *American Journal of Perinatology* 15:63–71.

Kanhai, H. H., de Haan, M., van Zanten, L. A., Geerinck-Vercammen, C., van der Ploeg, H. M., and Gravenhorst, J. B. 1994. Follow-up of pregnancies, infants, and families after multifetal pregnancy reduction. *Fertility and Sterility* 62:955–959.

Schreiner-Engel, P., Walther, V. N., Mindes, J., Lynch, L., and Berkowitz, R. L. 1995. First-trimester multifetal pregnancy reduction: Acute and persistent psychological reactions. *American Journal of Obstetrics and Gynecology* 172:541–547.

Couples Who Choose Embryo Donation

Sehnert, B., and Chetkowski, R. J. 1998. Secondary donation of frozen embryos is more common after pregnancy initiation with donated eggs than after in vitro fertilization-embryo transfer and gamete intrafallopian transfer. *Fertility and Sterility* 69:350–352.

Success Rate of Natural Cycle IVF

Zayed, F., Lenton, E. A., and Cooke, I. D. 1997. Natural cycle in-vitro fertilization in couples with unexplained infertility: Impact of various factors on outcome. *Human Reproduction* 12:2402–2407.

17. Having a Child through Donor Insemination

History of Donor Insemination

Kovacs, G. T., Mushin, D., Kane, H., and Baker, H. W. G. 1993. A controlled study of the psychosocial development of children conceived following insemination with donor semen. *Human Reproduction* 8:788–790.

Baker, D. J., and Paterson, M. A. 1995. Marketed sperm: Use and regulation in the United States. *Fertility and Sterility* 63:947–952.

1987 Survey

U.S. Office of Technology and Assessment. 1988. *Artificial Insemination: Practice in the United States.* Washington, D.C.: U.S. Government Printing Office.

ASRM Guidelines for Gamete Donation

1998. Guidelines for Gamete and Embryo Donation. *Fertility and Sterility* 70 (Suppl. 3):1S–13S.

HIV and Donor Insemination

Wortley, P. M., Hammett, T. A., and Fleming, P. L. 1998. Donor insemination and human immunodeficiency virus transmission. *Obstetrics and Gynecology* 91:515–518.

Linden, J. V., and Centola, G. 1997. Editorial: New American Association of Tissue Banks standards for semen banking. *Fertility and Sterility* 68:597–600.

Genetic Testing and Sperm Banks

Conrad, E. A., Fine, B., Hecht, B. R., and Pergament, E. 1996. Current practices of commercial cryobanks in screening prospective donors for genetic disease and reproductive risk. *International Journal of Fertility* 41:298–303.

Sperm Donation around the World

Meirow, D., and Schenker, J. G. 1997. Reproductive health care policies around the world: The current status of sperm donation in assisted reproduction technology: Ethical and legal considerations. *Journal of Assisted Reproduction and Genetics* 14:133–138.

Finances as Factor in the Choice to Use Donor Insemination

Schover, L. R., Thomas, A. J., Miller, K. F., Falcone, T., Attaran, M., and Goldberg, J. 1997. Preferences for intracytoplasmic sperm injection (ICSI) versus donor insemination (DI) in severe male factor infertility: A preliminary report. *Human Reproduction* 11:2461–2464.

Genetic Risk and the Choice of Infertility Treatment

Schover, L. R., Thomas A. J., Falcone, T., Attaran, M., and Goldberg, J. 1998. Attitudes about genetic risk of couples undergoing in-vitro fertilization. *Human Reproduction* 13:862–866.

Men with Vasectomies More Accepting of Donor Insemination

Nachtigall, R. D., Tshann, J. M., Quiroga, S. S., Pitcher, L., and Becker, G. 1997. Stigma, disclosure, and family functioning among parents of children conceived through donor insemination. *Fertility and Sterility* 68:83–89.

Barriers to Adoption

Chippindale-Bakker, V., and Foster, L. 1996. Adoption in the 1990s: Sociodemographic determinants of biological parents choosing adoption. *Child Welfare* 74:337–355.

Bachrach, C. A., Stolley, K. S., and London, K. A. 1992. Relinquishment of premarital births: Evidence from national survey data. *Family Planning Perspectives* 24:27–32, 48.

1994. Rethinking the choice to have children: When, how, and whether or not to bear children. *American Behavioral Scientist* 37:1058–1073.

Stigma Attached to Donor Insemination

Nachtigall, R. D., Tshann, J. M., Quiroga, S. S., Pitcher, L., and Becker, G. 1997. Stigma, disclosure, and family functioning among parents of children conceived through donor insemination. *Fertility and Sterility* 68:83–89.

Braverman, A. M., and Corson, S. L. 1995. Factors related to preferences in gamete donor sources. *Fertility and Sterility* 63:543–549.

A Survey of Men's and Women's Attitudes to Donor Insemination

Braverman, A. M., and Corson, S. L. 1995. Factors related to preferences in gamete donor sources. *Fertility and Sterility* 63:543–549.

Religious Views on Donor Insemination

Mor-Yosef, S., and Schenker, J. G. 1995. Sperm donation in Israel. *Human Reproduction* 10:965–967.

Study in Four European Countries

Golombok, S., Brewaeys, A., Cook, R., Giavazzi, M. T., Guerra, D., Mantovani, A., van Hall, E., Crosignani, P. G., and Dexeus, S. 1996. The European study of assisted reproduction families: Family functioning and child development. *Human Reproduction* 11:2324–2331.

Wives Tend to Underestimate Husband's Approval of Donor Insemination

Gillett, W. R., Daniels, K. R., and Herbison, G. P. 1996. Feelings of couples who have had a child by donor insemination: The degree of congruence. *Journal of Psychosomatic Obstetrics and Gynecology* 17:135–142.

Feelings about Donor Insemination Become More Positive
Daniels, K. R., Gillett, W. R., and Herbison, G. P. 1996. Successful donor insemination and its impact on recipients. *Journal of Psychosomatic Obstetrics and Gynecology* 17:129–134.

Marital Satisfaction in Donor Insemination
Schover, L. R., Collins, R. L., and Richards, S. 1992. Psychological aspects of donor insemination: Evaluation and follow-up of recipient couples. *Fertility and Sterility* 57:583–590.

Attitudes about Using Known Donors
Braverman, A. M., and Corson, S. L. 1995. Factors related to preferences in gamete donor sources. *Fertility and Sterility* 63:543–549.

Purdie, A., Peek, J. C., Irwin, R., Ellis, J., Graham, F. M., and Fisher, P. R. 1992. Identifiable semen donors—attitudes of donors and recipient couples. *New Zealand Medical Journal* 105:927–928.

Statistics on Egg Donation
Society for Assisted Reproductive Technology and the American Society for Reproductive Medicine. 1996. Assisted reproductive technology in the United States and Canada: 1994 results generated from the American Society for Reproductive Medicine/Society for Assisted Reproductive Technology Registry. *Fertility and Sterility* 66:697–705.

More Openness in Telling Children of Egg Donation
Pettee, D., and Weckstein, L. N. 1993. A survey of parental attitudes toward oocyte donation. *Human Reproduction* 11:1963–1965.

The Majority of Families Do Not Tell Child about Donor Insemination
Klock, S. 1997. The controversy surrounding privacy or disclosure among donor gamete recipients. *Journal of Assisted Reproduction and Genetics* 14:378–380.

Schover, L. R., Collins, R., and Richards, S. 1992. Psychological aspects of donor insemination: Evaluation and follow-up of recipient couples. *Fertility and Sterility* 57:583–590.

News Story on Donor Offspring
20/20 Transcripts: Faceless, nameless fathers: Donor offspring search for clues about their dads. January 19, 1998. http://archive.abcnews.com/onair/2...ml_files/transcripts/nmg0119a.html.

Recent Research on Children's Ideas about Heredity
Solomon, G. E., Johnson, S. C., Zaitchik, D., and Carey, S. 1996. Like father, like son: Young children's understanding of how and why offspring resemble their parents. *Child Development* 67:151–171.

Johnson, S. C., and Solomon, G. E. 1997. Why dogs have puppies and cats have kittens: The role of birth in young children's understanding of biological origins. *Child Development* 68:404–419.

No Relationship of Decision to Tell and Bonding

Nachtigall, R. D., Tshann, J. M., Quiroga, S. S., Pitcher, L., and Becker, G. 1997. Stigma, disclosure, and family functioning among parents of children conceived through donor insemination. *Fertility and Sterility* 68:83–89.

Regrets about Telling Others about Donor Insemination

Klock, S. 1997. The controversy surrounding privacy or disclosure among donor gamete recipients. *Journal of Assisted Reproduction and Genetics* 14:378–380.

18. The Pursuit of Paternity

Infidelity during Women's Fertile Times

Baker, R. R., and Bellis, M. A. 1995. *Human Sperm Competition: Copulation, Masturbation and Infidelity.* London: Chapman and Hall.

The Theory of Parental Investment

Trivers, R. L. 1972. Parental investment and sexual selection. In *Sexual Selection and the Descent of Man,* edited by B. Campbell. Chicago: Aldine, 1871–1971.

McDonald-Pavelka, M. S. 1995. Sexual nature: What can we learn from a cross-species perspective? In *Sexual Nature, Sexual Culture,* edited by P. R. Abramson and S. D. Pinkerton. Chicago: University of Chicago Press, 17–35.

Anthropological Studies of Mating in Different Cultures

Fisher, H. E. 1992. *Anatomy of Love: The Natural History of Monogamy, Adultery, and Divorce.* New York: W. W. Norton.

Gender Differences in Acceptance of Options to Treat Male Infertility

Schover, L. R., Thomas, A. J., Miller, K. F., Falcone, T., Attaran, M., and Goldberg, J. 1997. Preferences for intracytoplasmic sperm injection (ICSI) versus donor insemination (DI) in severe male factor infertility: A preliminary report. *Human Reproduction* 11:2461–2464.

The Value of Children

Murray, T. H. 1996. *The Worth of a Child.* Berkeley: University of California Press.

19. The Female Side of Male Infertility

Greater Distress in Infertile Women Than Men

Morrow, K. A., Thoreson, R. W., and Penney, L. L. 1995. Predictors of psychological distress among infertility clinic patients. *Journal of Consulting and Clinical Psychology* 63:163–167.

Wright, J., Duchesne, C., Sabourin, S., Bissonnette, F., Benoit, J., and Girard, Y. 1991. Psychosocial distress and infertility: Men and women respond differently. *Fertility and Sterility* 55:100–108.

Myers, M. F. 1990. Male gender-related issues in reproduction and technology. In *Psychiatric Aspects of Reproductive Technology,* edited by N. L. Stotland. Washington, D.C.: American Psychiatric Press, 25–35.

Women More Depressed with Failed IVF

Baram, D., Tourtelot, E., Muechler, E., and Huang, K. 1988. Psychosocial adjustment following unsuccessful in vitro fertilization. *Journal of Psychosomatic Obstetrics and Gynecology* 9:181–190.

Newton, C. R., Hearn, M. T., and Yuzpe, A. A. 1990. Psychological assessment and follow-up after in vitro fertilization: Assessing the impact of failure. *Fertility and Sterility* 54:879–886.

Men are Less Likely to Take Care of Preventive Health than Women

Hourani, L. L., and LaFleur, B. 1995. Predictors of gender differences in sunscreen use and screening outcome among skin cancer screening participants. *Journal of Behavioral Medicine* 18:461–477.

Myers, R. E., Ross, E., Jepson, C., Wolf, T., Balshem, A., Millner, L., and Leventhal, H. 1994. Modeling adherence to colorectal cancer screening. *Preventive Medicine* 23:142–151.

Men Are More Apt to Use Avoidance to Cope with Health Problems

Miller, S. M., Rodoletz, M., Schroeder, C. M., Mangan, C. E., and Sedlacek, T. V. 1996. Applications of the monitoring process model to coping with severe long-term medical threats. *Health Psychology* 15:216–225.

22. The Spiritual and Ethical Side of Infertility

Schwartz, A. 1994. A rabbinic response to infertility. In *Be Fruitful and Multiply: Fertility Therapy and the Jewish Tradition,* edited by R. V. Grazi. Jerusalem: Genesis Jerusalem Press.

23. Robbing Paul to Pay Peter: The Economics of Male Infertility

State Laws on Infertility Insurance

American Society for Reproductive Medicine web site, http://www.asrm.com/patient/insur.html. Accessed September 8, 1998.

Infertility Costs in Massachusetts

Griffin, M., and Panak, W. F. 1998. The economic cost of infertility-related services: An examination of the Massachusetts infertility insurance mandate. *Fertility and Sterility* 70:22–29.

Costs of Raising a Child

Johnston, P. I. 1997. *Launching a Baby's Adoption: Practical Strategies for Parents and Professionals*. Indianapolis: Perspectives Press.

Cost-effectiveness of Superovulation

Rammer, E., and Friedrich, F. 1998. The effectiveness of intrauterine insemination in couples with sterility due to male infertility with and without a woman's hormone factor. *Fertility and Sterility* 69:31–36.

Van Voorhis, B. J., Sparks, A. E., Allen, B. D., Stovall, D. W., Syrop, C. H., and Chapler, F. K. 1997. Cost-effectiveness of infertility treatments: A cohort study. *Fertility and Sterility* 67:830–836.

Zayed, F., Lenton, E. A., and Cooke, I. D. 1997. Comparison between stimulated in-vitro fertilization and stimulated intrauterine insemination for the treatment of unexplained and mild male factor infertility. *Human Reproduction* 12:2408–2413.

Vasectomy Reversal versus IVF-ICSI

Donovan, J. F., DiBaise, M., Sparks, A. E., Kessler, J., and Sandlow, J. I. 1998. Comparison of microscopic epididymal sperm aspiration and intracytoplasmic sperm injection/in-vitro fertilization with repeat microscopic reconstruction following vasectomy: Is second attempt vas reversal worth the effort? *Human Reproduction* 13:387–393.

Kolettis, P. N., and Thomas, A. J., Jr. 1997. Vasoepididymostomy for vasectomy reversal: A critical assessment in the era of intracytoplasmic sperm injection. *Journal of Urology* 158:467–470.

Pavlovich, C. P., and Schlegel, P. N. 1997. Fertility options after vasectomy: A cost-effectiveness analysis. *Fertility and Sterility* 67:133–141.

Cost-effectiveness of Treating Varicoceles

Schlegel, P. N. 1997. Is assisted reproduction the optimal treatment for varicocele-associated male infertility? A cost-effectiveness analysis. *Urology* 49:83–90.

Guaranteed IVF Success

Andereck, W. S., Thomasma, D. C., Goldworth, A., and Kushner, T. 1998. The ethics of guaranteeing patient outcomes. *Fertility and Sterility* 70:416–421.

Ethics Committee of the American Society for Reproductive Medicine. 1998. Shared-risk or refund programs in assisted reproduction. *Fertility and Sterility* 70:414–415.

24. Choosing to Adopt a Child

Statistics on Number of Adoptive Families

Adoptive Families of America. 1998. URL: http://www.cyfc.umn.edu.adoptinfo/afa.htm#fact. Accessed July 29.

Statistics on Numbers of Yearly Adoptions in the United States

Adoptive Families of America. 1998. Guide to adoption. URL: http://www.cyfc.umn. edu.adoptinfo/afa.htm#fact. Accessed July 29.

Adoption Network. 1998. Adoption: Frequently asked questions: How many adoptions are accomplished each year? URL: http://207.226.25.92/about/html.body_ faq6.html. Accessed July 19.

Numbers of International Adoptions

International Adoption Statistics. 1998. Cradle adoptions. URL: http//www.cradle. org/Statistics/internat.html. Accessed July 22.

Insurance Agency that Offers Adoption Insurance

MBO Insurance Brokers. 1998. URL: http://www.adopting.org/mbo.html. Accessed July 29.

Putative Father Registries

National Adoption Information Clearinghouse. 1998. Legal issues of independent adoption. URL: http://www.adoption.com/library/articles/legal.shtml. Accessed July 22.

Costs of Adoption

Mooney, Mary Lib. 1998. *The Adoption Agency Guide.* URL: http://www.adoption-assist.com/aag/dave.htm. National Council for Adoption. Accessed July 27.

Statistics on Birth Rates in 1996

U.S. Department of Health and Human Services. 1998. Report of final natality statistics, 1996. Vol. 46, no. 11 (suppl). PHS 98-1120. URL: http://www.cdc.gov/ nchswww/releases/98news/natal96.htm. Accessed July 27.

Caucasian Women Who Give Up Infants for Adoption

Bachrach, C. A., Stolley, K. S., and London, K. A. 1992. Relinquishment of premarital births: Evidence from national survey data. *Family Planning Perspectives* 24:27–32.

Transracial Adoption

Vroegh, K. S. 1997. Transracial adoptees: Developmental status after 17 years. *American Journal of Orthopsychiatry* 67:568–575.

Hollingsworth, L. D. 1998. Promoting same-race adoption for children of color. *Social Work* 43:104–116.

Children in the Foster Care System

Adoptive Families of America. 1998. URL: http://www.cyfc.umn.edu.adoptinfo/afa. htm#fact. Accessed July 29.

Failures of Special Needs Adoptions

Adoptive Families of America's Guide to Adoption. 1998. URL: http://www.cyfc.umn. edu.Adoptinfo/adoptionguide.html. Accessed July 29.

Birth Mother Contact

Lee, J. C., and Waite, J. A. 1997. Open adoption and adoptive mothers: Attitudes toward birth mothers, adopted children, and parenting. *American Journal of Orthopsychiatry* 67:576–584.

Open Adoption and Birth Mothers

Blanton, T. l., and Deschner, J. 1990. Biological mothers' grief: The postadoptive experience in open versus confidential adoption. *Child Welfare* 69:525–535.

Open Adoption and Adoptive Parents

Wrobel, G. M., Ayers-Lopez, S., Grotevant, H. D., McRoy, R. G., and Friedrick, M. 1996. Openness in adoption and the level of child participation. *Child Development* 67:2358–2374.

Berry, M. 1993. Adoptive parents' perceptions of, and comfort with, open adoption. *Child Welfare* 72:231–253.

Searching for Birth Parents

Sachdev, P. 1989. The triangle of fears: Fallacies and facts. *Child Welfare* 68:491–503.

Estimates of Numbers who Search

National Adoption Information Clearinghouse. 1998. Searching for birth relatives. URL: http://www.adoption.com/library/articles/search.shtml. Accessed July 22.

Reunions with Adoptive Parents

Campbell, L. H., Silverman, P. R., and Patti, P. B. 1991. Reunions between adoptees and birth parents: The adoptees' experience. *Social Work* 36:329–335.

25. Living without Children

Study of the Impact of Having a Child on Infertile Couples

Abbey, A., Andres, F. M., and Halman, L. J. 1994. Infertility and parenthood: Does becoming a parent increase well-being? *Journal of Consulting and Clinical Psychology* 62:398–403.

Rituals to Mark the End of Infertility Treatment

Zoldbrod, A. P. 1993. *Men, Women, and Infertility: Intervention and Treatment Strategies.* New York: Lexington Books, 97–98.

Index